ALCOHOL
POISONING MORTALITY
IN FOUR NORDIC COUNTRIES

Distributors:

AKATEEMINEN KIRJAKAUPPA,
Keskuskatu 1, 00100 Helsinki 10, Finland

RUTGERS UNIVERSITY CENTER OF ALCOHOL STUDIES,
Smithers Hall, New Brunswick, New Jersey 08903, U.S.A.

THE FINNISH FOUNDATION FOR ALCOHOL STUDIES,
ALKOHOLITUTKIMUSSÄÄTIÖ
Kalevankatu 12, 00100 Helsinki 10, Finland

ISBN 951-9191-47-X (C)
ISBN 951-9191-48-8 (P)

Printed in Finland
by Aurasen Kirjapaino
Forssa 1977

ALCOHOL POISONING MORTALITY

IN FOUR NORDIC COUNTRIES

BY

KARI POIKOLAINEN

ALCOHOL RESEARCH IN THE NORTHERN COUNTRIES
THE FINNISH FOUNDATION FOR ALCOHOL STUDIES
VOLUME 28

Translated

by

EVA PALMGREN

Sunt aliquot quoque res quarum unam dicere causam
non satis est, verum pluris, unde una tamen sit;
corpus ut exanimum siquod procul ipse iacere
conspicias hominis, fit ut omnis dicere causas
conveniat leti, dicatur ut illius una;
nam neque eum ferro nec frigore vincere possis
interiisse neque a morbo neque forte veneno,
verum aliquid genere esse ex hoc quod contigit ei
scimus. item in multis hoc rebus dicere habemus.

LUCRETIUS: *De Rerum Natura,* VI, 703—711.

CONTENTS

LIST OF FIGURES

LIST OF TABLES

ABBREVIATIONS, DEFINITIONS AND SYMBOLS

Abbreviations

a	all cases in Sweden
ADH	alcohol dehydrogenase
ICD	International Statistical Classification of Diseases, Injuries, and Causes of Death
NAD	nicotinamide-adenine dinucleotide, oxidized form
NADH	nicotinamide-adenine dinucleotide, reduced form
o/oo	per mille (per thousand)
s	Swedes only
WHO	World Health Organization

Quantity of alcohol

Quantities of alcohol have been reported as grams of 100 per cent ethanol. If in the original article alcohol consumption has been expressed as volume units, the latter have been multiplied by 0.79 – the specific gravity of ethanol – to obtain the corresponding magnitude in weight units. If unspecified, the reported concentrations have been assumed to be given as volume per volume. Ounces that have not been specified have been presumed to be U.S. fluid ounces (29.57 ml).

Statistical symbols

df	degrees of freedom
p	probability of error when rejecting the null hypothesis (p-value, level of significance)
x	test not applicable, because over 20 per cent of cell frequencies less than five

Symbols of numerical observations

–	no observations
0	less than half the unit shown
..	data not available
e	estimate based on extrapolation from a sample

Units of alcohol concentration

The magnitudes of alcohol concentration are given as per mille (per thousand). In Denmark, Finland and Norway the concentrations have been measured as weight per weight units, in Sweden as weight per volume units. The discrepancy between these two modes of measurement is negligible, since the specific gravity of body fluids and tissues is close to unity (Wallgren and Barry 1970, 31).

I
INTRODUCTION

According to the official statistics, there are considerable differences in mortality from alcohol poisoning between the different Nordic countries. The order with regard to the death rates for 1960—1967, in descending order, was Finland, Norway, Sweden, Denmark (Bruun 1972, 122). In contrast, the total alcohol consumption and the mortality from liver cirrhosis were clearly higher in Denmark and Sweden than in Norway and Finland (Bruun 1972, 57 and 115). A similar trend in the death rates for alcohol poisoning might have been anticipated.

The decision to undertake this study on the causes of the differences in mortality from alcohol poisoning was prompted by the above-mentioned discrepancies. The purpose of the study was to identify those factors to which the variations in alcohol poisoning mortality may be attributed, to analyse their implications for the differences between the four Nordic countries in question*, and to assess the deviations of the statistically recorded mortality from the actual mortality.

Comparative approach

Inter-country comparisons often provide descriptive information constituting a basis for etiological studies. Moreover, the purpose of comparative investigations often involves making causal inferences. Despite the complex demands this may make on research, an attempt is generally made in comparisons to arrive at conclusions that concern etiological relations. Verification of the causal hypotheses is facilitated if the selection of the observation units, i.e. the areas to be studied, can be carried out so as to simulate designs used in experimental research. In practice, however, this is often possible only to a limited extent due to the difficulties connected with the collection of material; in-

* Iceland was excluded from the comparison because the number of cases was small in this country. The annual number of accidental poisoning deaths (AE 140 in the ICD) varied from one to six during the years 1961—1970.

stead, comparisons have to be based on historical-administrative units such as states or provinces. This method is appropriate for descriptive purposes, but it does not fulfil the demands of an analytical investigation equally well (Allardt 1975, 57–58).

The reason why it is judicious to compare the Nordic countries lies in the fact that a strategy of maximal similarity can be applied (Allardt 1975, 55). Some of the factors potentially explaining differences may be omitted from consideration because of their similarity in the countries concerned, which resemble each other closely with regard to cultural, social and physical characteristics. In this investigation the treatment of the victims of alcohol poisoning was one such factor, since the principles of treatment and the criteria for admission to hospital have a markedly levelling effect owing to the similarity of medical standards and organized health care in the Nordic countries. Moreover, with the exception of Finland, these countries proved similar with regard to morbidity as measured by the interview technique (Allardt 1975, 94) and mortality estimated by official statistical data (Bolander 1971); the Finnish figures for both morbidity and mortality were higher. Impairment of general physical fitness due to illness might be assumed to provide some explanation for the differences in mortality from alcohol poisoning between the Nordic countries. However, morbidity does not seem to explain the differences observed between Norway, Sweden and Denmark. Thus, general morbidity does not seem to be a factor of importance in this connection.

In studies concerned with inter-country differences, comparability is essential. It is often taken for granted, and the correlations between the dependent and independent variables are analysed on the basis of the available material. Consequently, it is generally difficult to draw any definite conclusions, and the reliability of the results is open to criticism. Comparability in studies on mortality is influenced by (1) thoroughness in tracing the causes of deaths and (2) diagnostic practice. Variations in thoroughness may be assumed to impair reliability, as random errors are likely to ensue and the correlations found are thus underestimated. On the other hand, diagnostic variations in the countries compared may cause systematic errors as regards the mortality from the causes of death in question.

Factors influencing the differences in mortality from alcohol poisoning

In a study of the differences in mortality from alcohol poisoning between the Nordic countries, the factors influencing comparability play an essential role. The thoroughness in tracing causes of death varies from one country to the next, and as a rule the body of data on deaths suspected to be due to alcohol poisoning remains scanty unless special investigations are undertaken (Alha and Isotalo 1964).

Diagnostic practice is an important potential source of error in inter-country comparisons of mortality from alcohol poisoning, since opinions differ with regard to the causal order of the various abnormalities preceding death and with regard to the diagnostic criteria. Death statistics are based on the cause that initiates the process terminating in death, and post-mortem examination may reveal several potentially lethal abnormalities. It can be stated what diseases the patient suffered from or died with, but it is difficult to establish which of them he died of. It has been advocated that alcoholism has been arbitrarily indicated as the underlying cause of death in many cases in which coincident pathologies are present (Bruun et al. 1975, 20). For this reason an analysis of the diagnostic criteria of death from alcohol poisoning and of the causal relationships in cases with a fatal outcome constitutes an important part of the present investigation. The effect of the possible differences in diagnostic practice on the mortality rates for alcohol poisoning is evaluated with regard to alcoholism and also with regard to certain conditions for which a high alcohol consumption is a risk factor.

Theoretical considerations and empirical data indicate that the higher the per capita consumption in a population, the greater is the prevalence of heavy drinkers (Bruun et al. 1975, 30–39). It might be assumed from the data on alcohol consumption (Svendsen 1976) that heavy drinking was most frequent in Denmark, followed by Sweden, Finland and Norway, in that order, in 1967–1971. Alcohol poisoning mortality rates in these countries might be expected to correlate with the frequencies of heavy drinkers. However, the amount of alcohol consumed is not necessarily related to the risk of death from alcohol poisoning, since the amount consumed per day may be considerable although the concentration of ethanol in the blood never rises to a level that would entail serious functional disturbances, let alone lethal consequences. Therefore, the relationship between alcohol consumption and alcohol poisoning mortality is not likely to be straightforward.

Death from alcohol poisoning results when the ethanol concentration in the brain tissue rises to a level that causes paralysis of the respiratory centre. Violent drinking aimed at rapidly producing a state of deep intoxication is thus a factor that enhances the risk of alcohol poisoning and is also the cause of death if the poisoning is sufficiently severe. It was therefore assumed that the differences in mortality from alcohol poisoning in the Nordic countries are attributable to differences in the frequency of uncontrolled drinking.

The validity of the above-mentioned assumption was tested by ascertaining whether any features implicating heavy drinking could be observed in the material of fatal alcohol poisonings. In evaluating the occurrence of uncontrolled drinking the following questions were posed: (1) Do high death rates for alcohol poisoning occur in sparsely inhabited provinces in which the alcohol consumption is low, (2) is an accumulation of deaths from alcohol poisoning observable in the context of those holidays on which alcohol is generally consumed in large quantities, (3) are there any inter-country differences in the post-mortem blood ethanol concentrations of the victims of alcohol poisoning, (4) do the groups of lethally alcohol poisoned in the various countries differ in relation to the frequency of Skid Row alcoholism, (5) are any differences observable in those who have died of alcohol poisoning with regard to the frequency of pathological changes known to be associated with the use of alcohol, and (6) what inter-country differences in mortality from alcohol poisoning can be demonstrated if only cases selected by criteria defined on the basis of the literature are accepted as deaths from this cause.

An analysis of these aspects cannot provide any final answer to the question of whether the inter-country differences in mortality from alcohol poisoning are attributable to differences in the frequency of uncontrolled drinking, since only indirect evidence can be studied. However, when all the results are considered, conclusions may be drawn which provide a fairly reliable answer.

The risk of death from alcohol poisoning clearly depends on the rate of drinking. In addition, the risk may be influenced by certain factors modifying the resistance of the organism to the lethal effects of alcohol. It has been suggested that coronary heart disease (Alha 1970a) and age (Saldeen and Johansson 1967) are such factors, but so far these hypotheses have not been proved. It should be borne in mind that heavy use of alcohol sustained over a long period is often associated with a decline in social status and a change in the drinker's way of life characterized by vagrancy, poor eating habits, poor hygiene and the use of cheap substitute alcohols. This way of life may in turn be associated with morbidity or other incapacitating factors, which may enhance the risk of death from alcohol poisoning.

Purpose of the investigation

The purpose of this investigation was

(1) to describe the earlier drinking habits, way of life, morbidity and demographic characteristics of persons who have died of alcohol poisoning,

(2) to clarify whether any differences exist between the Nordic countries with regard to thoroughness in tracing causes of death, what these differences are due to, and whether they influence the differences in mortality from alcohol poisoning,

(3) to find out whether cases which in Finland would be attributed to alcohol poisoning are differently classified in the other Nordic countries,

(4) to ascertain whether the inter-Nordic differences in mortality from alcohol poisoning are attributable to different drinking habits, and
(5) to clarify whether the observed statistical inter-Nordic differences in mortality from alcohol poisoning reflect real differences and, if not, to what extent they deviate from these.

II
PATHOGENESIS AND CRITERIA OF ALCOHOL POISONING DEATHS

The literature dealing with the pathogenesis and criteria of deaths from alcohol poisoning and the adequacy of the criteria are examined. Moreover, the factors influencing the values for blood ethanol concentration – the most important criterion of alcohol poisoning – are discussed.

Pathogenesis of deaths from alcohol poisoning

A state of severe intoxication may be life-threatening in many ways. After a long period of drinking, sudden abstinence may precipitate a fatal attack of delirium. An intoxicated person may fall in the snow and freeze to death or die in a hot sauna or be burnt to death. An alcoholic may carelessly drink a whole bottle of toxic industrial alcohol containing e.g. methanol, isopropanol or ethylene glycol. A mentally distressed person seeking relief from anxiety may use a quantity of alcohol which in combination with drugs paralyses his bodily functions owing to the synergism of the substances. A drunk person may aspirate vomit or take a posture which obstructs the airways and thus causes suffocation.

In all these instances intoxication plays an important, although not necessarily decisive role in the cause-and-effect chain terminating in death. Apart from the various alcohol-related hazards, the intoxication as such may be lethal. In this case the effect of alcohol on the central nervous system is thought to be responsible for paralysis of the cells of the respiratory centre, resulting in cessation of the vital functions owing to oxygen deficiency.

It has been suggested that mechanisms other than paralysis of the respiratory centre may be contributory causes of death from alcohol poisoning. Mention has been made of (1) cerebral fat embolism, (2) tissue hypoxia resulting from the aggregation of blood cells and (3) hypoglycaemia. The possibility of deaths from alcohol poisoning being attributable to these factors will be discussed later. The question here is whether the phenomena mentioned as causative are necessary consequences of deep intoxication and whether alone they suffice to account for a fatal outcome.

Respiratory failure

The view that the paralysing effect of ethanol on the respiratory centre may be the cause of death is based on animal experiments and clinical observations. Klingman and Haag (1958) reported that dogs infused with ethanol intravenously at the rate of about 2 grams per kg of body weight per hour died after four hours. After intravenous administration, death always seemed to be due to failure of the respiratory function. When a dose of about 10 grams ethanol per kg of body weight was administered into the stomach, about 65 per cent of the dogs survived for a maximum of 12 hours and death apparently resulted from respiratory failure. In those dogs who survived for over 12 hours, death was preceded by a progressive fall in blood pressure caused by circulatory failure.

The cardiac and circulatory failure associated with alcohol poisoning slowly terminating in death appears to be primarily due to depression of the respiratory function. Loomis (1952) reported that the cardiac function ceased in some dogs given about 24 grams ethanol (weights of dogs not stated) while weak respiration was still observable. The failure of the heart was attributed to hypoxia resulting from ethanol-induced paralysis of the respiratory centre and to the increased toxic effect of ethanol on the myocardium associated with hypoxia. Polaczek-Kornecki et al. (1971) observed no direct effect on the myocardium after intravenous administration of 7—10 grams ethanol per kg body weight to dogs. When alcohol poisoning took a slow lethal course, the failure of cardiac function was apparently due to hypoxia and a diminishing venous return. The authors considered the pathophysiological condition primary normovolaemic toxic shock; no features typical of cardiogenic shock were noticed.

The mechanism of ethanol-induced paralysis of the respiratory centre is not clearly understood. It has been suggested that ethanol paralyses the neural control area, which normally maintains an excitatory state in the respiratory centre (Rosenstein et al. 1968).

Fat embolism

Fat embolism in brain, heart and lungs has been adduced as a possible explanation of the sudden death of chronic alcoholics (Durlacher et al. 1954, Lynch et al. 1959, Prokop 1966, 516). It is believed that fat emboli originate from fat cysts in the liver cells. It has also been suggested that emboli may be formed in hyperlipaemic states in connection with the destabilization of emulgated fat (Thaler 1963, Bschor 1963). This hypothesis has not been proved.

Durlacher et al. (1954) observed massive fat emboli in five out of 25 bodies showing fatty liver attributed to alcohol use. Fat embolism was noticed by Lynch et al. (1959) in 31 out of 40 cases of fatty liver. The number of emboli in the individual cases was markedly lower than that generally seen in connection with fractures, whereas Durlacher et al. (1954) found about the same number as in fracture cases. Lynch et al. (1959) thought that some cause other than fat embolism was the underlying cause of death in most cases. Both these series were short and controls were not used.

Pulmonary fat emboli are a common autopsy finding in subjects who have died of trauma without having shown any noteworthy clinical signs of disturbed pulmonary function (Sevitt 1960). Therefore, the above results permit no conclusions with regard to causal relationships, bearing in mind moreover that in experimental investigations on the rabbit fat emboli have been demonstrated in considerable numbers within 18 hours from death (Allardyce 1971).

Aggregation of blood cells

The ingestion of even moderate amounts of alcohol induces aggregation of red blood cells. The degree of aggregation correlates positively with the blood ethanol concentration (Forsander and Suomalainen 1955). Moskow et al. (1968) proposed a mechanism for explaining the tissue damage due to ethanol. It was suggested that the aggregation of red blood cells is followed by a retardation of the blood flow, stasis, transudation of the plasma proteins to the interstitial spaces, oedema, disturbed tissue oxygenation, oxygen deficiency and cell damage.

Moskow et al. (1968) examined microscopically the aggregation of red blood cells in the retinal blood vessels in 36 alcoholics admitted for treatment while drunk. The higher the ethanol concentration at the time of examination, the more conspicuous was the aggregation. Massive aggregation, retardation of the blood flow and stasis of blood vessels were observed in those showing the highest blood ethanol concentration (2.6—3.3 per mille). The correlation observed was inter-individual, and the relationship between the degree of aggregation and the amount of alcohol ingested before admission to hospital was not assessed. The results do not prove that the blood ethanol concentration and the degree of aggregation correlate intra-individually during acute intoxication.

Pennington and Knisely (1973) studied the aggregation of red blood cells in deaths from alcohol poisoning by administering lethal doses of ethanol to rabbits pretreated with heparin and to non-treated rabbits. The pretreated rabbits survived significantly longer after intake of the lethal dose than the untreated rabbits. The aggregation of red blood cells was significantly slighter and occurred later in the heparin-treated rabbits than in the untreated group. No appreciable differences in blood ethanol concentration measured at the moment of death were observed. The results indicate that aggregation of the red blood cells after the administration of a lethal dose of ethanol may accelerate death. They do not prove that the aggregation as such is a mechanism responsible for death from alcohol poisoning.

Hypoglycaemia

Under certain circumstances, fatal hypoglycaemia may result from the use of alcohol. The subject has been reviewed by Arky (1971), and Arky and Freinkel (1969). More than 125 cases of ethanol-induced hypoglycaemia have been described in 32 different publications (Arky and Freinkel 1969). The majority of subjects developing hypoglycaemia have been undernourished persons or chronic alcoholics, but a reduction of the blood glucose concentration has also been observed in healthy, well-nourished children and adolescents subjected to the influence of ethanol and fasting (Arky 1971, 212).

After acute administration of ethanol, hyperglycaemia develops when the accelerated adrenalin secretion causes a breakdown of glycogen in the liver (Forsander et al. 1958). Stored glycogen seems to counteract hypoglycaemia, since the development of experimental hypoglycaemia presupposes a fast of 24—36 hours in normal test subjects and fasting for a shorter period in patients whose glycogen reserve is low (Freinkel et al. 1965). The hypoglycaemia that develops after a fast of 16—24 hours is slight in patients anaesthetized with ethanol or with methohexital (Dundee et al. 1972). By contrast, after a 74-hour fast test subjects given ethanol revealed a considerable degree of hypoglycaemia (Arky and Freinkel 1969). A positive correlation has been found between the frequency and degree of experimental ethanol-induced hypoglycaemia and the duration of the preceding fast (Freinkel et al. 1963).

The oxidation of ethanol in the liver raises the intrahepatic NADH/NAD ratio, resulting in a retardation of the gluconeogenesis (Madison et al. 1967). Ethanol thus inhibits the production of glucose in the liver. On the other hand, it also may reduce the peripheral utilization of glucose (Madison 1968). This phenomenon may explain the fact that hypoglycaemia is seldom seen in alcoholics (Madison 1968).

In this connection it cannot be decided whether undernourishment alone is a sufficient prerequisite for the development of ethanol-induced hypoglycaemia, or whether a certain lability of the glucose homeostasis is also required. However, ethanol alone will not produce this condition. Therefore, hypoglycaemia cannot be considered a typical consequence of ethanol poisoning.

On analysing fatal cases of ethanol poisoning, ethanol-induced hypoglycaemia does not seem to be a mechanism of crucial importance, although it may be fatal in connection with prolonged fasting. In malnourished chronic alcoholics, fasting may also cause ketoacidosis (Levy et al. 1973), which becomes manifest after the disappearance of ethanol from the organism. The lethality of this state remains to be evaluated.

Criteria of death from alcohol poisoning

No anatomical or histological abnormalities typical of alcohol poisoning are known (Linck 1953, Edmondson et al. 1956, Saldeen and Johansson 1967). The establishing of the cause of death is mainly based on toxicological studies, primarily determinations of the blood alcohol concentration. At the same time attention is paid to preceding events, autopsy and histological findings, and other toxicological analyses possibly performed. When considering alcohol poisoning as a cause of death, the question as to what is the best indicator of the lethal effect of alcohol is a fundamental one.

The lethal dose of ethanol

An excessive amount of ethanol is lethal. However, the lethal dose cannot be clearly defined. Its size depends on many factors, of which body size, fluid volume, absorption of the ethanol from the intestinal tract, strength of the beverage ingested, the drinking rhythm, ethanol oxidation rate and the time spent on drinking are the most important. Edmondson et al. (1956) stated that a dose of about 250—500 grams of 100 per cent ethanol, or about 3—7 grams per kg of body weight, rapidly consumed is lethal. According to Linck (1950), about 200—250 grams of 100 per cent alcohol, or about 2.0—3.5 grams per kg of body weight, is a lethal dose for adult men. Widmark (1933) calculated the theoretical lethal dose as ethanol absorbed by the organism in males and females of different sizes. The mean lethal dose for persons weighing 70 kg was 238 grams for males and 193 grams for females.

The lethal concentration of ethanol

In general, the blood ethanol concentration and the physiological effects of alcohol correlate positively. The correlation is not perfect, since other factors — above all tolerance — are also involved. Tolerance to many of the pharmacological effects of alcohol may develop, but it has been stated that no evidence of the development of tolerance to the lethal ethanol concentration has been produced (Koppanyi et al. 1961). On the other hand, Gormsen's (1973) estimates of the lethal ethanol concentration as well as the high blood ethanol concentrations (p. 32) noted by Majchrowicz and Mendelson (1971) indicate that such tolerance may develop. This question deserves further clarification.

On the basis of what is known about the pathogenesis of deaths from alcohol poisoning, the ethanol concentration in the nerve cells of the respiratory centre seems to be the best indicator of the lethal ethanol concentration. Since it is impossible in practice to measure this concentration, it seems advisable to assess the degree to which the blood ethanol concentration approximates to the ethanol concentration in the brain cells of the respiratory centre.

During the absorption stage the alcohol concentration in the tissues is mainly determined by arterial blood flow (Haggard et al. 1940). However, an equilibrium between the arterial blood and the brain tissue appears to be rapidly attained. Fischer and Wallgren (1957) observed that in dogs it took on average 85 seconds for an equilibrium to be established between the brain tissue and the blood. Scherrer-Etienne and Posternak (1963) found that the ethanol concentration in the cat brain depended on the blood flow during the first minute from infusion, but an equilibrium between the blood and the grey matter of the brain was attained within a few minutes.

The parameters relating to the lethal concentration of blood ethanol have been determined in many animal species (Wallgren and Barry 1970, 55—60). However, the experience, acquired in animal experiments, of the biological variation in dose-response relationships cannot be applied to humans. Estimation of the variations in the lethal effect of ethanol in man, therefore, constitutes a problem. It is difficult to form a confident opinion on the cumulative relative frequency distribution of the lethal blood ethanol concentration or to calculate the median lethal blood ethanol concentration. Knowledge of the fatal concentration in humans is derived mainly from clinical case reports and pathologic-toxicological investigations.

The average lethal blood ethanol concentration in adult humans has been estimated at about 4 per mille (Forney and Hughes 1968, 4), 5 per mille (Widmark 1933, Wallgren and Barry 1970, 58), 5—6 per mille (Kaye and Haag 1957), 5.5 per mille (Himwich 1957, French 1971) or 6—9 per mille (Forney and Harger 1965). Widmark (1933) stated that less than 4 per mille is seldom fatal, while over 6 per mille is a concentration that few people survive. The lowest blood ethanol concentration capable of killing adult humans has been estimated at 3 per mille (Wallgren and Barry 1970, 58) or somewhat over (Jarosch 1975) or 3.5 per mille (French 1971, Himwich 1957).

Nordic medicolegal experts have given somewhat lower estimates of the lethal concentration than the authors mentioned above. Saldeen and Johansson (1967) stated that the blood ethanol concentration in those dying from alcohol poisoning varies between 3.5 and 4.5 per mille. Gormsen (1973) regards 2.5 to

3.0 per mille as a concentration that may kill persons unaccustomed to drinking, while the lethal level for habitual drinkers is 3.0 to 3.5 per mille. A similar view has been expressed by Lundevall (1973), who stated that over 3.5 per mille is generally, though not invariably, a lethal concentration. The two last-mentioned authors drew attention to the fact that intoxicated persons have been reported to survive a blood ethanol concentration of 4 to 5 per mille. The lower estimates given by medicolegal experts may be attributed to the occurrence of lower blood ethanol levels after death than before. In addition, it seems possible that medicolegal series are more representative of the general population than clinical series since the former are more likely to include both high and low lethal concentrations.

The blood ethanol concentrations measured post mortem in cases of alcohol poisoning are on average clearly lower than the maximum values obtaned before death. The average post-mortem blood ethanol concentration in victims of fatal alcohol poisoning is about 3.5 to 4.5 per mille (Table 1). The variation of the post-mortem concentrations is wide, the range being from 0.50 to 6.55 per mille (Table 1).

Table 1. Post-mortem blood ethanol concentration in alcohol poisoning deaths

Time of investigation	Number of cases	Blood ethanol concentration (per mille)			Authors and year of publication
		Arithmetic mean	Median	Range of variation	
1939–1943	16	3.58	3.58	2.34–5.20	Linck 1948/49
1948–1955	94	..	4.60	1.80–6.00	Kaye and Haag 1957
1957–1965	5	4.00	..	2.60–5.60	Saldeen and Johansson 1967
1959–1968	113	..	..	0.50–6.55	Marcinkowski and Przybylski 1974*
1969–1972	7	4.47	4.50	3.50–5.14	Jarosch 1975
1976	242	3.57	..	1.84–6.01	Alha, personal communication**

* Aspiration of gastric contents into the lower respiratory tract was a contributory cause of death in some cases (number not indicated).

** Cases investigated at the Division of Forensic Chemistry, Department of Forensic Medicine, University of Helsinki.

The highest blood ethanol concentrations noted in living individuals

Information on the highest tolerated blood ethanol concentrations may be obtained from three different sources. These are (1) medicolegal examinations of drivers suspected of being under the influence of drink, (2) reports of cases treated for alcohol poisoning and (3) experimental investigations concerned with the blood alcohol concentration during drinking sessions.

Studies of drivers suspected of being under the influence of drink have shown that about one per cent had a blood ethanol concentration in excess of 3 per mille (Table 2). The high tolerance sometimes developed by alcoholics is exemplified by the fact that some of those examined had been capable of driving despite being extremely intoxicated. In a German report, among drivers subjected to examination for some reason other than a road accident a blood ethanol concentration of 4.00—4.59 per mille was noted in eight among 34 883 drivers (Häussler and Mallach 1973). Concentrations approaching the lethal level are thus relatively infrequent in series selected on the basis of a suspicion of drunkenness.

Very high ethanol concentrations have sometimes been noted in patients admitted to hospital for alcohol poisoning. The highest concentration from which a patient has ever recovered at the Hesperia Hospital in Helsinki was 7.58 per

Table 2. Percentage of subjects showing a blood ethanol concentration of over three per mille in series of drivers examined for alcohol intoxication

Time of investi-gation	Number of cases	Cases with over three per mille Per cent	Country	Authors and year of publication
1960—1971	34 883	1.4	Federal Republic of Germany	Häussler and Mallach 1973
1962	6 686	0.3	Denmark	Gürtler and Lund 1966
..	868	1.0	Sweden	Andréasson and Bonnichsen 1964
1965—1969	6 839	0.6	Finland	Penttilä et al. 1972
1966—1971	7 127	1.4	Federal Republic of Germany	Kossman 1972
1972	11 653	1.0	Finland	Alha 1974

mille (Forsman et al. 1976). Furthermore, many patients with an ethanol concentration of over 5 per mille have been successfully treated. According to a report from the U.S.A., a 23-year-old woman survived poisoning with an ethanol concentration of 7.8 per mille (Hammond et al. 1973).

In a group of 10 alcoholics given 400 grams 100 per cent ethanol in the form of whisky for five days the maximum blood alcohol concentration was 3.5 per mille and the average was about 2.5 per mille (Mendelson and La Dou 1964, 20). When 19 alcoholics were allowed to drink whisky or brandy of their own free will for 10 to 14 days in an amount corresponding to a maximum of 370 grams 100 per cent ethanol, the maximum blood ethanol concentration varied between 4.1 and 5.0 per mille* (Majchrowicz and Mendelson 1971). These findings suggest that the concentration resulting from voluntary drinking may sometimes approach the lethal level in habitual drinkers.

Factors influencing the values for the post-mortem ethanol concentration

When diagnosing deaths from alcohol poisoning, the degree to which the blood ethanol concentration measured post mortem corresponds to the maximum ante-mortem level is of fundamental importance. To facilitate evaluation of the significance of blood ethanol values obtained post mortem in cases of alcohol poisoning, those factors will be analysed which influence the ethanol concentration from the time when the maximum value is arrived at to the time when the postmortal level is determined. These factors are (1) antemortal changes in the blood ethanol concentration, (2) postmortal changes in the blood ethanol concentration and (3) errors connected with the measurement of these concentrations.

Antemortal changes in the blood ethanol concentration

The ethanol concentration in the blood often falls considerably during the interval between the point of time when the maximum is attained and the moment of death. The decline can be assessed if the length of this interval and the decline rate are known. The estimate obtained is unbiased provided that an equilibrium in ethanol diffusion exists between the blood and the tissues. In this case the decline rate of the blood ethanol concentration is the same as

* In this ethically dubious experiment the concentration exceeded 5 per mille in some cases, but the exact value is not indicated.

the elimination rate. The latter depends on both the oxidation rate and the excretion rate of ethanol. Ingested ethanol is oxidized in the organism at an even rate (Mellanby 1919)*. Since the excretion rate is slight compared with the oxidation rate, the elimination rate is practically constant. The antemortal decline of the blood ethanol concentration is the product of the elimination rate and the time lapse.

If a large volume of ethanol is rapidly ingested, the diffusion rate of ethanol from the blood into the tissues may be higher than the rate of the reverse process even after the peak in blood ethanol concentration has been attained. In this case the decline in blood ethanol is initially larger than that indicated by the elimination rate and it is, therefore, overestimated by the method described above. It is important to bear this in mind when the empirical results obtained on the parameters determining the blood ethanol concentration are surveyed in the following. The purpose of the review is to arrive at a crude estimate of the antemortal decline in blood ethanol.

The precise distribution of the length of the interval between the point of time when the maximum blood ethanol concentration is reached and the moment of death from alcohol poisoning is not known. However, some values have been published. The interval was estimated by Edmondson et al. (1956) at about 5 to 12 hours, by Alha and Isotalo (1964) at about 6 to 12 hours. In a report on 94 deaths from alcohol poisoning, Kaye and Haag (1957) estimated the interval at one to 16 hours. Linck (1950) gave an estimate of 2 to 12 hours in a series of 36 cases. On the basis of the data reported by Linck, the average interval may be calculated at about 6.5 hours. That very long intervals may occur appears from the reports on two boys, aged 16 and 15, who died of alcohol poisoning 20 and 22–24 hours, respectively, after they had stopped drinking (Rodier and Gentile 1952, Regus 1937). As a rule, the maximum blood ethanol concentration is attained within two hours, usually within one hour, from the discontinuation of drinking (Zink and Reinhardt 1975).

The means for the blood ethanol elimination rate in human experiments have ranged from 0.119 to 0.412 per mille per hour (Table 3). Much of the variation seems to be due to differences in drinking habits between the

---

* On the basis of a case of severe alcohol poisoning Hammond et al. (1973) alleged that the decrease of the blood ethanol concentration is an exponential function of time. Their observations seem, however, to be accounted for by changes in the patient's fluid balance (Mezey 1974). On the other hand, if the blood ethanol concentration is very low, the elimination actually changes from linear to exponential (Widmark 1932, 44). The concentration at which the elimination is altered is apparently the same as the Michaelis constant of the hepatic ADH catalyzing the ethanol-acetaldehyde reaction, or about 0.025–0.1 per mille (Wallgren and Barry 1970, 95 and 100, Lieber 1975).

Table 3. Rate of blood ethanol elimination in abstainers, moderate users of alcohol and alcoholics

Alcohol use and sex of study group	Number of cases	Elimination rate (per mille per hour)		Authors and year of publication
		Arithmetic mean	Standard deviation	
Moderate users, male	19	0.119	0.019	Jokipii 1951, 48
Total abstainers, male	9	0.125	0.014	Goldberg 1943, 104
Over 14 days' abstinence, males	109	0.129	0.024	Alha 1951, 44–46
Normal females and males	39	0.130	0.039	Reisby 1971
Moderate users, female	23	0.132	0.020	Jokipii 1951, 48
Moderate users, male	16	0.138	0.021	Goldberg 1943, 104
Heavy users, male	14	0.143	0.019	Goldberg 1943, 104
Alcoholics, 3 weeks after a drinking bout, male	6	0.156	0.016	Shah et al. 1972*
Moderate users	12	0.158	..	Pawan 1972
Alcoholics, after a drinking bout, male	25	0.164	0.027	Mezey and Tobon 1971*
Alcoholics, after 15–30 days' abstinence, male	23	0.186	0.082	Ugarte et al. 1972**
Alcoholics, one week after a drinking bout, male	6	0.245	0.038	Shah et al. 1972*
Alcoholics, after 6–14 days' abstinence, male	20	0.256	0.112	Ugarte et al. 1972**
Alcoholics, after a drinking bout, male	19	0.272	0.030	Majchrowicz and Mendelson 1971
Alcoholics who had ingested alcohol during the preceding 24 hours, male	17	0.356	0.103	Ugarte et al. 1972**
Alcoholics, after a drinking bout, male and female	18	0.412	0.079	Kater et al. 1969*

* Serum values divided by 1.20.

** Standard deviations calculated as the product of standard error and the square root of the number of cases.

experimental groups. The mean for abstainers or moderate users is 0.119–0.158, the mean for alcoholics who have abstained for at least some days is 0.156–0.256, and the mean of the values obtained for alcoholics just after a drinking bout is 0.272–0.412 per mille per hour (Table 3). On the other hand, the standard deviations for the elimination rate indicate that the intra-group variance also is considerable. It may thus be concluded that the more abundant and recent the use of alcohol, the greater is the elimination rate likely to be, although wide individual differences occur.

There is good reason to be cautious with regard to the great variation in the values for the elimination rate. The values obtained may differ considerably from each other depending on which values are chosen for determining the elimination rate (Sjöberg 1964). As pointed out by Karu (1975), high values for the constant of elimination rate may be attributable to the fact that a linear elimination pattern has been fitted to measurements in part obtained before the diffusion equilibrium is established. This may apply, for instance, to an investigation in which a record-high value for the elimination rate was reported (Kater et al. 1969), since the linear regression coefficient was calculated using as the first observation a measurement taken 60 minutes after the cessation of alcohol ingestion. However, irrespective of this source of error, it seems likely that alcohol consumption increases the value for the elimination rate, as this value was also found to decrease when repeated measurements were performed on alcoholics one, two and three weeks after a sustained period of drinking (Shah et al. 1972).

Postmortal changes in the blood ethanol concentration

It has been stated that the postmortal diffusion of unabsorbed alcohol from the stomach into the blood may distort the view taken of the premortal ethanol concentration (Huber 1943, Gifford and Turkel 1956, Bowden and McCallum 1949). This conclusion has been drawn from studies in which ethanol was instilled into the stomach in dead bodies and the ethanol concentration was measured in different parts of the body. However, it has been shown that while large amounts of ethanol diffuse into the pericardial and pleural fluids, only small amounts appear in the blood (Plueckhahn and Ballard 1967). Moreover it is noteworthy that the amount of ingested alcohol remaining in the stomach at the moment of death is usually small. In autopsy series alcohol has been found to constitute at most 5 per cent of the gastric fluid and in general much less (Plueckhahn 1968).

It has been alleged that the ethanol concentrations measured in heart blood are too high owing to postmortal diffusion, and that blood samples should therefore be drawn from the femoral vein (Gifford and Turkel 1956). However, erroneously high values in heart blood may be due to the admixture of pericardial fluid into the blood (Plueckhahn 1968). Comparisons of the ethanol concentrations measured in blood samples obtained from intact ventricles and from the femoral vein have not revealed any statistically significant differences (Plueckhahn and Ballard 1967, Falconer and Falconer 1973). In conclusion, it may be stated that the diffusion of ethanol does not significantly alter the blood ethanol concentration, if the blood has been collected in an approved manner and no substantial changes due to putrefaction are observed (Plueckhahn 1968).

The formation of ethanol certainly caused by putrefaction has been observed after an interval of at least 48 hours after death (Wolthers 1958). Results not influenced by postmortal putrefaction have been obtained even three to four days after death. The ethanol concentration resulting from putrefaction seldom exceeds 0.5 per mille (Weiler and Reh 1974), though it may occasionally approach 1 per mille (Alha, personal communication 1977). There are clear variations between different parts of the vascular system in the concentration of ethanol formation after death (Wolthers 1958, Falconer and Falconer 1973).

The alcohols formed by the putrefaction process may be bacterial or fungal metabolic products. Certain bacteria are capable of fermenting carbohydrates, with a resultant formation of ethanol and higher aliphatic alcohols. Fungi may also dissolve the glucose present in the body and produce alcohols (Plueckhahn 1967). In one or two days considerable quantities of ethanol may be produced by micro-organisms in blood stored at room temperature. The resulting concentration usually reaches its maximum within 10 to 14 days, after which it slowly falls (Plueckhahn 1967). Concentrations of about 0.5 per mille have been found in infected animal tissues within three days after death (Davis 1973). On the other hand, the ethanol concentration in the blood may decrease after death as a result of enzymatic activity. Oxidation of ethanol is theoretically possible as long as pyruvate is formed by glycolysis, when NADH is oxidized to NAD (Kalant 1968).

The principal factor responsible for infection is contamination in the autopsy room. In contrast, the interval between death and autopsy, the duration of hospital care and the basic disease do not seem to be major risk factors in this respect (O'Toole et al. 1965).

The addition of sodium fluoride in a 1 per cent solution inhibits the formation of alcohol in blood samples stored for 10 days at room temperature (Plueckhahn 1968). If fluoride and oxalate are added, no notable change in ethanol concentration occurs for at least 10 months in blood samples stored at 5°C or lower temperatures (Sunshine and Hodnett 1971). The blood ethanol concentration undergoes no noteworthy changes in bodies kept for an average of 32 hours under appropriate conditions in a cool mortuary (Francisco and Baldwin 1972). In conclusion, it may be established that the postmortal blood ethanol values in general correspond to the concentration at the time of death, provided that no essential changes due to putrefaction are observed in the body, that the blood sample has been drawn within 48 hours from death, and that the sample is appropriately stored (Wolthers 1958, Plueckhahn 1967).

Measurement errors

The dichromate method is based on the capacity of dichromate in sulphuric acid to oxidize ethanol, which can be measured fluorometrically, titrimetrically or photometrically (Sunshine and Hodnett 1971). The method is not specific for ethanol; other volatile organic substances such as some aldehydes, esters, methanol and the higher aliphatic alcohols oxidize in the same way (Kalant 1968). If any of these substances are present in the sample, the value for ethanol obtained by the dichromate method will be too high. The sensitivity of the method may be increased by chemical elimination of the substances responsible for the error. The steam distillation method (Sunshine and Hodnett 1971) utilizes mercuric oxide for the elimination of aldehydes and ketones from the distillate. The best modifications of the dichromate method have a standard deviation of about 0.06 per mille (Kalant 1968).

The enzymatic method of ethanol determination utilizes a reaction in which ethanol is oxidized by the action of ADH into acetaldehyde at the same time as NAD is reduced. A quantitative estimate of ethanol is obtained by measuring the amount of NADH formed photometrically (Sunshine and Hodnett 1971). The accuracy of the enzymatic method is greater than that of the dichromate method. The standard deviation is about 0.5—1.5 per cent of the actual ethanol concentration (Kalant 1968). With regard to ethanol, the enzymatic method is more specific than the dichromate method, although not absolutely specific (Wallgren and Barry 1970, 34). Gas chromatography is the most specific method for the determination of ethanol, but its accuracy does not differ from that of the enzymatic method. The standard deviation of liquid gas chromatography has been indicated at one per cent of the actual ethanol concentration within the range of 0.15—2.6 per mille (Cravey and Jain 1974).

III
MATERIAL AND METHODS

This investigation is based on official cause-of-death and vital statistics. In the analysis of some questions the statistical data could be used as such. In addition, it was used as a basis of sampling for the central part of the investigation, for which the material was obtained from the records of cause-of-death inquiries. The systems of cause-of-death inquiries were analysed on the basis of the pertinent laws, statutes and written principles of application.

Official statistics

The statistical data used in this investigation was obtained from the cause-of-death and vital statistics published in the Nordic countries or from unpublished sources (p. 165). In the cause-of-death statistics the cases are classified by the underlying cause of death (p. 124) and they are published in this form. In addition to the underlying cause of death, the death certificate may contain notes on other, contributory causes of death and on the immediate cause of death which is due to the underlying cause. Theoretically, analysis of the contributory causes of death is a better approach to the study of alcohol poisoning mortality than analysis limited to the statistics based on the underlying cause of death. However, in the Nordic countries data on contributory causes of death have only been published in Sweden and Denmark. The reasons for indicating or not indicating contributory causes of death in the death certificate and the differences in registration practice are not known. In the present investigation analysis was therefore confined to the underlying causes of death.

Statutes concerning inquiries into the cause of death

The relationship between the system of inquiring into the cause of death and the mortality from alcohol poisoning as recorded in the official statistics was assessed by comparing the legal principles of cause-of-death inquiries in the different Nordic countries. This analysis was based on the laws and statutes relating to cause-of-death examinations and their interpretation in the literature. Since the majority of alcohol poisoning deaths falls within the field of the medicolegal systems of cause-of-death inquiries, the regulations governing these and their various modes of application in practice are dealt with separately (Appendix 1).

Material obtained from records of cause-of-death inquiries

Most of the results of the present investigation are based on data obtained from the records of cause-of-death inquiries. The sources from which the information was collected consisted of death certificates, records of police inquiries and autopsy records as well as reports on chemical and histological examinations connected with autopsy. The collection of this data will be described in detail, since it constitutes the body of the present material.

The first step was to study chronological series of deaths in the official Nordic cause-of-death statistics. These series were used as a basis for selecting groups suitable for comparison. A clear variation in the number of recorded alcohol poisoning deaths was observed both between the Nordic countries and between different years in the same country. Except in Denmark, mortality from alcohol poisoning increased from the early 1960's to the early 1970's. In the Swedish chronological series of deaths from alcohol poisoning and alcoholism surprising variations were seen, which seemed to cancel each other out. The assumption was made that a proportion of cases which in Finland would have been labelled as death from alcohol poisoning, in Sweden had been diagnosed as death from alcoholism. It was decided to test this hypothesis by comparing the cases recorded in Sweden as deaths from alcoholism with the cases diagnosed in Sweden and Finland as deaths from alcohol poisoning and with the cases recorded in Finland as deaths from alcoholism. In both Norway and Denmark the number of deaths attributed to alcoholism was so small that the alcohol poisoning mortality rates cannot have been appreciably influenced even if the diagnostic difference mentioned above existed. The Norwegian and Danish cases of death from alcoholism were therefore not included in the material.

The material consists of cases belonging to six different groups: alcohol poisoning deaths in the four Nordic countries and deaths from alcoholism in Finland and Sweden. To reduce chance variations one hundred was set as the minimum number of cases in each group.

Selection of cases and sampling

The study groups assembled primarily from the statistics for 1967—1971 varied considerably in size. In some instances it was considered unnecessary to study the whole group; a sample was therefore used.

In *Denmark* only 87 deaths from alcohol poisoning had been statistically recorded in 1967—1971, and the material was therefore supplemented by the deaths that had occurred in 1966. According to the statistics, the total number of deaths in 1966—1971 was 109. However, two death certificates were not found, and one case had been erroneously recorded as death from alcohol poisoning, although the actual cause was suicide by parathion. When this case was excluded, the Danish group of alcohol poisonings consisted of 106 cases.

In *Finland* deaths exceeded the number considered adequate and systematic sampling was therefore applied. Of the alcohol poisoning deaths every third case was selected from lists of names arranged in alphabetical order, and from this lot every eighth case was omitted. The first case for every year was selected at random. The study group thus obtained consisted of 328 cases. Of the deaths from alcoholism every second case was selected and every sixth of these cases was omitted. In the group of deaths from alcoholism four cases had been erroneously coded; alcoholism had not been indicated as the underlying cause of death*. After exclusion of these cases the Finnish study group of deaths from alcoholism consisted of 118 cases.

In *Norway* the death certificates for all those who had died of alcohol poisoning in 1967—1971 were collected and studied. The statistically recorded cases numbered 237, but as one more death certificate was found, the Norwegian group of alcohol poisoning deaths consisted of 238 cases.

In *Sweden* all alcohol poisoning deaths from 1967—1971 were included in the study group. According to the official statistics they numbered 328. However, in three cases the underlying cause of death had been erroneously coded**. After exclusion of these cases the Swedish group of alcohol poisoning deaths consisted of 325 cases. The selection of deaths from alcoholism was performed by sampling. This was applied to the years 1969—1971 only, since in this way the time spent on collecting death certificates could be reduced. Every fifth case was selected from annual lists arranged by year of birth. The sample thus obtained consisted of 115 cases.

The representativeness of the samples with regard to age was assessed by comparing them to the total material of officially recorded cases. The age dis-

---

* The true underlying causes of death were *necrosis totalis acuta pancreatis, insufficientia cordis acuta, pancreatitis acuta haemorrhagica* and *pancreatitis haemorrhagica.*

** The underlying causes of death were *diabetes mellitus, ethylene glycol poisoning* and *trichloroethylene poisoning.*

tribution of the samples differed only slightly from the distribution anticipated on the basis of the official statistics. The differences in age distribution between the samples and the data base (Table 4) were not statistically significant as is shown by the Chi-square goodness of fit test (p = .251–.965). The groups obtained by systematic sampling methods were thus representative of the base population with regard to age.

Collection of records of cause-of-death inquiries

The data obtained from the death certificates was supplemented by information collected from the records of cause-of-death examinations kept at medicolegal institutions and hospitals, from the cause-of-death archives of the Finnish National Board of Health and from the archives of the Norwegian Medicolegal Commission.

Denmark. The records of all cases were placed at the author's disposal by the medicolegal institutions. The death certificates showed that no examinations had been performed in hospitals in any case of alcohol poisoning.

Table 4. Compatibility of age distribution in samples and total groups of males who died of alcohol poisoning or alcoholism during the time of investigation

	Alcohol poisoning		Alcoholism			
	Finland		Finland		Sweden[a]	
Age group (years)	Observed number of cases	Expected number of cases	Observed number of cases	Expected number of cases	Observed number of cases	Expected number of cases
–24	7	8.6	} 8	} 7.7	} 10	} 8.0
25–29	6	9.8				
30–34	11	16.6				
35–39	40	47.3	7	9.5	8	6.5
40–44	57	52.5	25	26.8	5	10.3
45–49	63	51.3	26	23.7	14	13.6
50–54	41	41.1	12	13.4	19	16.4
55–59	36	32.5	14	11.2	16	17.6
60–64	31	25.5	12	12.1	11	10.9
65–69	} 15	} 21.5	} 8	} 7.4	9	8.2
70–					7	7.4
Total	307	306.7	112	111.8	99	98.9
p-value	.251		.965		.835	
df	9		7		8	

Chi-square goodness of fit test

Finland. The records were found in the archives of the National Board of Health for all cases except three of those in which the death certificate stated that autopsy had been performed.

Norway. According to the death certificates, autopsy had been performed in 151 out of 238 cases. The autopsy reports on 125 cases were obtained. Thus, 17 per cent of all autopsy reports were apparently missing, although it should be noted that the statements on the death certificates were often vague on this point, or the forms contained no paragraph relating to autopsy.

Sweden. According to the death certificates autopsy had been performed in 288 out of 325 cases. The autopsy reports on 258 cases were obtained, and the proportion of missing reports was thus 10 per cent. According to the death certificates, autopsy had been performed on 95 subjects who had died of alcoholism. The report was obtained in 92 cases; the proportion of missing cases was thus 3 per cent. The reasons why autopsy reports were not obtainable in Sweden were (a) that part of the records kept in the archives of the National Institute of Forensic Medicine in Gothenburg were out on loan and (b) that reports on only 52 out of 68 cases (76 per cent) autopsied in hospitals were obtained by mail.

Variables

The following paragraphs deal with those variables and classifications which proved most problematic. At the same time the reliability of the subject matter of the variables is discussed.

Country. Each country was given its own code. In addition, three groups were distinguished in Sweden: people born in Sweden, Finnish immigrants and immigrants from countries other than Finland. Among those who died of alcohol poisoning in Sweden in 1967—1971, 15 were Finnish immigrants and 6 were immigrants from other countries. Among those who had died of alcoholism, the corresponding numbers were 13 and one.

The results for Sweden were calculated either on the total study group (a) or on those deceased persons who were born in Sweden (s). The reason for this distinction was that some phenomena of interest were considered to be related to Swedish national characteristics, others to the character of Sweden as a state.

Province. For inter-country comparisons, information was collected with regard to the places of death or domicile. Initially the purpose was to record the province where the death *de facto* occurred for each of the deceased, as this was assumed to elucidate best the situation prevailing before death. However, for practical reasons the *de facto* province was codified only for the Finnish material. In order to reduce the burden of work the *de jure* place of domicile was recorded for the study groups from the other Nordic countries. This hardly reduces the reliability of inter-province comparisons of mortality, as migration due to morbidity caused by or related to the use of alcohol in all likelihood mostly occurs within provinces.

Place of death. The place of death was usually clearly indicated when police inquiries had been made. In contrast, when such inquiries had not been made, the place of death was often either vaguely indicated or not indicated at all. This applies in particular to Norway, where information on the place of death was lacking in 31 per cent of the cases of alcohol poisoning.

Earlier use of alcohol. If possible, the use of alcohol preceding the drinking occasion leading to death was assessed by a variable classified as follows: (1) temperance, (2) moderate use, (3) heavy use and (4) consumption at the Skid Row level. With regard to the first three groups, classification was based on alcohol consumption alone. Consumption at the Skid Row* level was assumed if the records gave evidence not only of heavy use of alcohol but also of a definite decline in social status, lack of a permanent job and fixed address, or membership of a typical alcoholic community. The classification was based on information obtained from official records. Deep intoxication once a week or a daily consumption exceeding 80 grams 100 per cent ethanol was considered as heavy use of alcohol. However, only in a fraction of the cases was it possible to assess the consumption with any degree of accuracy. In the majority of cases the estimates had to be based on the impressions received by those who had written the official reports. The value of the results is reduced by the fact that no information at all was obtained in a large proportion of the cases. Information on previous alcohol consumption was not obtained in 16 per cent of those who had died of alcohol poisoning in Denmark, 49 per cent of the Finnish material, 77 per cent of the Norwegian material and 44 per cent of the Swedish alcohol poisoning cases. With regard to deaths from alcoholism, information was lacking in 13 per cent of the Finnish material and 21 per cent of the Swedish material.

The different Nordic countries seemed to reveal little discrepancy in their methods of collecting information on autopsied cases. This enhances the comparability of the data of this study. Minor differences in the frequency of chemical and histological special examinations were noticed, but it is not likely that these were of fundamental importance. The data collected by the police in the different Nordic countries was also comparable. In contrast, a wide discrepancy between the study groups in the frequency of autopsied cases gave cause for concern. The autopsy ratio of those cases whose autopsy records were obtained for this study to all investigated alcohol poisoning deaths was 97 per cent in Finland, 79 per cent in Sweden, 58 per cent in Denmark and 52 per cent in Norway.

* The most common form and spelling of the term Skid Row has been adopted in the text. According to Spradley (1970, 8), the original form is Skid Road.

Data processing

The data collected for analysis was coded on forms and transferred to punched cards and thence on to magnetic tape for computer processing. The punched cards were subjected to check-up perforation.

Punching errors were checked in two ways. When the data written in numerical form was inspected by eye, a number of errors in the matrix were detected and corrected. Logically impossible observations were brought out by calculating the minimum and maximum values of the variables and by cross-tabulations of the variables.

Demographic characteristics of the subjects studied

Sex

The majority of those whose death was attributed to alcohol poisoning or alcoholism were men. The proportion of men among those who had died of alcohol poisoning was highest in Finland (94 per cent), slightly lower in Norway and Sweden (89 per cent) and lowest in Denmark (75 per cent). The proportion of men among those who had died of alcoholism was 95 per cent in Finland and 87 per cent in Sweden. It is striking that the proportion of men was so much lower in Denmark than in the other Scandinavian countries.

Marital status

Among those who had died of alcohol poisoning the proportion of divorced persons was clearly higher in Denmark than in the other Nordic countries (Table 5). The proportion of unmarried men was slightly greater among those who had died of alcohol poisoning than among those who had died of alcoholism. On comparing the distribution by marital status of the men who had died of alcohol poisoning or alcoholism to the corresponding distribution in the total male population over 15 years of age in the Nordic countries (Nordic Council 1972, 27), divorced men were found to be strongly overrepresented in the present material. Unmarried men and widowers were also clearly overrepresented, although not to the same extent as divorcees. Bearing in mind that the phenomenon is not attributable to age (Fig. 1), it may be concluded that unmarried and divorced men and widowers run a greater risk of dying from alcohol poisoning than married men.

Table 5. Marital status in the study groups

Marital status	Alcohol poisoning				Alcoholism	
	Denmark Per cent	Finland Per cent	Norway Per cent	Sweden[s] Per cent	Finland Per cent	Sweden[s] Per cent
Unmarried	31	37	38	35	43	38
Married	23	37	31	33	27	27
Divorced	36	20	20	28	27	26
Widow(er)	10	7	11	5	3	9
Total	100	101	100	101	100	100
Number of cases	106	328	235	304	117	100
No information	–	–	3	–	1	1

Age

The mean age of the men who had died of alcohol poisoning was lowest in Denmark and Finland, 48 years. The men who had died of alcohol poisoning in Norway and Sweden were slightly older; their mean age was 50 years in Norway and 49 years in Sweden. The mean age of those whose death was recorded as due to alcoholism was 49 years in Finland, 52 years in Sweden. The men who had died of alcoholism were thus somewhat older than the men who had died of alcohol poisoning in both Finland and Sweden. The mean ages of the women who had died of alcoholism or alcohol poisoning corresponded to a large extent to the mean ages of the men.

Statistical methods

Statistical methods serve to condense the data collected and to quantify the uncertainty of the inferences made. They are by and large a means of expressing the observations in a clear and intelligible form. Therefore, the methods used in this investigation will be described in the sections on methods and results in the chapters dealing with the various features of alcohol poisoning mortality. However, some general comments on the terminology and application of the methods seem to be appropriate in this context.

Two tests based on the chi-square distribution (Diem and Lentner 1973, 166–168) are used in this investigation. The *chi-square goodness of fit test* is used to measure the identity of the sample and the base population. The *chi-square contingency test* is used to calculate the statistical significance of the association between two cross-tabulated variables on the null hypothesis of complete independency. Both these test are always two-sided in this study. The p-values are calculated without the Yates' correction for continuity.

The differences between the groups of alcohol poisoning and alcoholism deaths in the different Nordic countries were tested using 2 x 2 contingency tables. Only the chi-square contingency test p-values are presented. The p-values are given to the third decimal to permit the evaluation of probabilities between and outside the usual .05, .01 and .001 levels of significance.

IV
STATISTICALLY RECORDED MORTALITY FROM ALCOHOL POISONING AND ALCOHOLISM IN THE NORDIC COUNTRIES – DIFFERENCES AND TRENDS

In a study concerned with the inter-Nordic differences in alcohol poisoning mortality the official statistics are a valuable source of information. The statistical data provides an avenue of approach for many questions: the extent to which the differences cannot be attributed to chance, the impact of the age structure on the differences, the stability of the differences from year to year, time trends of the mortality rates, and the death risk in different age groups. In attempting to elucidate these points by analysis of the statistical data, deaths from alcoholism were also considered, since it was presumed that there is a great resemblance between alcoholism and alcohol poisoning as causes of death.

Material and methods

The material consisted of the vital statistics for the Nordic countries from the years 1961–1973. In the death statistics the cases were classified by underlying cause of death in accordance with the international cause-of-death classification and by age and sex. The Seventh Revision of the International Classification (WHO 1957) was used before 1969; from this year onwards the Eighth Revision (WHO 1967) was used. The code number for alcohol poisoning was E 880 in the Seventh Revision and E 860 in the Eighth Revision; the corresponding codes for alcoholism were 322 and 303.

The effect of the age structure of the population was assessed by comparing the actual mortality rates with age-standardized values. The age-standardized death rates were obtained by adding together the age-specific mortality rates of the study population weighted by the relative size of the respective age groups of the standard population. The average for all the Nordic populations throughout the period 1961–1973 was used as the standard population.

The statistical significance of the differences between the mortality rates was estimated by comparing the 99 per cent confidence intervals of the rates determined by the Poisson distribution. The differences were considered statistically significant if the confidence intervals did not fall within the same magnitude. The Poisson model was chosen as the probability distribution because it is produced by random events occurring independently of each other in time when the period is long and the probability of the individual event is small (Remington and Schork 1970, 120—121). The 99 per cent confidence limits were obtained from exact iterative tables (Diem and Lentner 1973, 108 and 189).

Trends were demonstrated by calculating five-year moving averages for the age-standardized mortality rates. A chronological series composed of moving averages contains less variation than the actual chronological series and the trend is therefore more conspicuous (Spiegel 1961, 285—286). The drawback of this method is that the information obtained on the initial and final parts of the chronological series is missing when moving averages are used. By calculating the moving five-year averages for the period 1961—1973 the observations for the first two and last two years were lost.

Results

Mortality by sex in 1967—1971

Alcohol poisoning mortality was markedly higher in Finland than in the other Nordic countries during the period 1967—1971. The difference in male mortality was striking, but the alcohol poisoning mortality among females was also clearly higher in Finland (Table 6). The alcohol poisoning mortality in males in Finland was about 1 450 per cent higher than in Denmark, about 320 per cent higher than in Norway and about 520 per cent higher than in Sweden. The alcohol poisoning mortality in females in Finland was about 600 per cent higher than in Denmark, about 130 per cent higher than in Norway and about 250 per cent higher than in Sweden. All inter-country differences in male mortality were significant ($p < .01$). The mortality of Finnish females was significantly higher than the mortality of Danish, Norwegian and Swedish females ($p < .01$). There were no other significant differences in female mortality between the Nordic countries.

The age-standardized alcohol poisoning mortality rate was higher than the actual mortality rate in both sexes in Finland and in Danish females. In Swedish males, the age-standardized mortality rate was lower than the actual rate (Table 6). Howerer, the actual and age-standardized values did not deviate much from each other. The greatest deviation was noted for Finnish males, whose age-

Table 6. Actual and age-standardized alcohol poisoning mortality by sex in the Nordic countries 1967–1971

	Mortality (per one million person-years)			
	Denmark	Finland	Norway	Sweden
Males				
Actual mortality	6	93	22	15
Age-standardized	6	103	22	14
Females				
Actual mortality	1	7	3	2
Age-standardized	2	8	3	2

Table 7. Annual number of alcohol poisoning deaths by sex in the Nordic countries 1967–1971

	Denmark		Finland		Norway		Sweden	
Year	Males	Females	Males	Females	Males	Females	Males	Females
1967	9	4	213	10	27	6	77	6
1968	12	2	218	23	33	2	99	11
1969	14	6	187	16	44	4	15	3
1970	18	3	202	14	54	7	18	5
1971	16	3	215	16	53	7	84	10

standardized mortality rate was 11 per cent higher than the actual rate. The differences in age-standardized mortality rates between the countries were greater than the differences in the actual rates.

The annual number of males who had died of alcohol poisoning in 1967–1971 was about 200 in Finland, about 60 in Sweden, about 50 in Norway and about 14 in Denmark. In Sweden, the number of deaths varied greatly from year to year (Table 7). The number of females who had died of alcohol poisoning was in general under 10 in all the Scandinavian countries.

The inter-country differences in mortality from alcoholism did not parallel the differences in alcohol poisoning mortality. Mortality from alcoholism, both male and female, was highest in Sweden (Table 8). Male mortality from alcoholism in Sweden was about 850 per cent higher than in Denmark, about 65 per cent higher than in Finland and about 280 per cent higher than in Norway. Female mortality from alcoholism in Sweden was about 200 per cent higher than in Finland and about 500 per cent higher than in Norway. The inter-country differences were more conspicuous in males than in females. All the male mortality rates differed from each other to a significant extent ($p < .01$). Mortality from alcoholism was significantly greater in Swedish than in Danish, Norwegian and Finnish females ($p < .01$).

Table 8. Actual and age-standardized alcoholism mortality by sex in the Nordic countries 1967–1971

	Mortality (per one million person-years)			
	Denmark	Finland	Norway	Sweden
Males				
Actual mortality	4	23	10	38
Age-standardized	4	26	9	36
Females				
Actual mortality	0	1	2	6
Age-standardized	0	1	2	5

Table 9. Annual number of alcoholism deaths by sex in the Nordic countries 1967–1971

	Denmark		Finland		Norway		Sweden	
Year	Males	Females	Males	Females	Males	Females	Males	Females
1967	7	2	21	–	14	3	133	19
1968	6	–	36	1	16	3	133	11
1969	7	–	74	4	19	1	164	26
1970	8	2	64	5	18	5	193	31
1971	20	1	64	5	26	3	135	24

The age-standardized rates for mortality from alcoholism were lower than the actual rates for Swedish males and females and Norwegian males (Table 8). In contrast, in Finnish males the age-standardized mortality rate for alcoholism was higher than the actual rate. The inter-country differences in age-standardized mortality rates were smaller than the differences in actual rates, but the order between the countries was the same.

The annual number of males statistically recorded as dying from alcoholism in 1967–1971 was about 150 in Sweden, about 50 in Finland, about 20 in Norway and under 10 in Denmark (Table 9). The corresponding number of females was about 20 in Sweden, while only occasional cases had been annually recorded in Denmark, Finland and Norway.

Mortality by age groups in 1967–1971

A survey of alcohol poisoning mortality in 1967–1971 by five-year age groups showed that the peak in mortality was reached in Finland by males aged 45–54 years, in Norway by those aged 45–49 and in Sweden by the age group 50–59 (Fig. 1). No clear peak in alcohol poisoning mortality was observed in Danish

Figure 1. Age-specific alcohol poisoning and alcoholism mortality in males in Denmark, Finland, Norway and Sweden 1967–1971

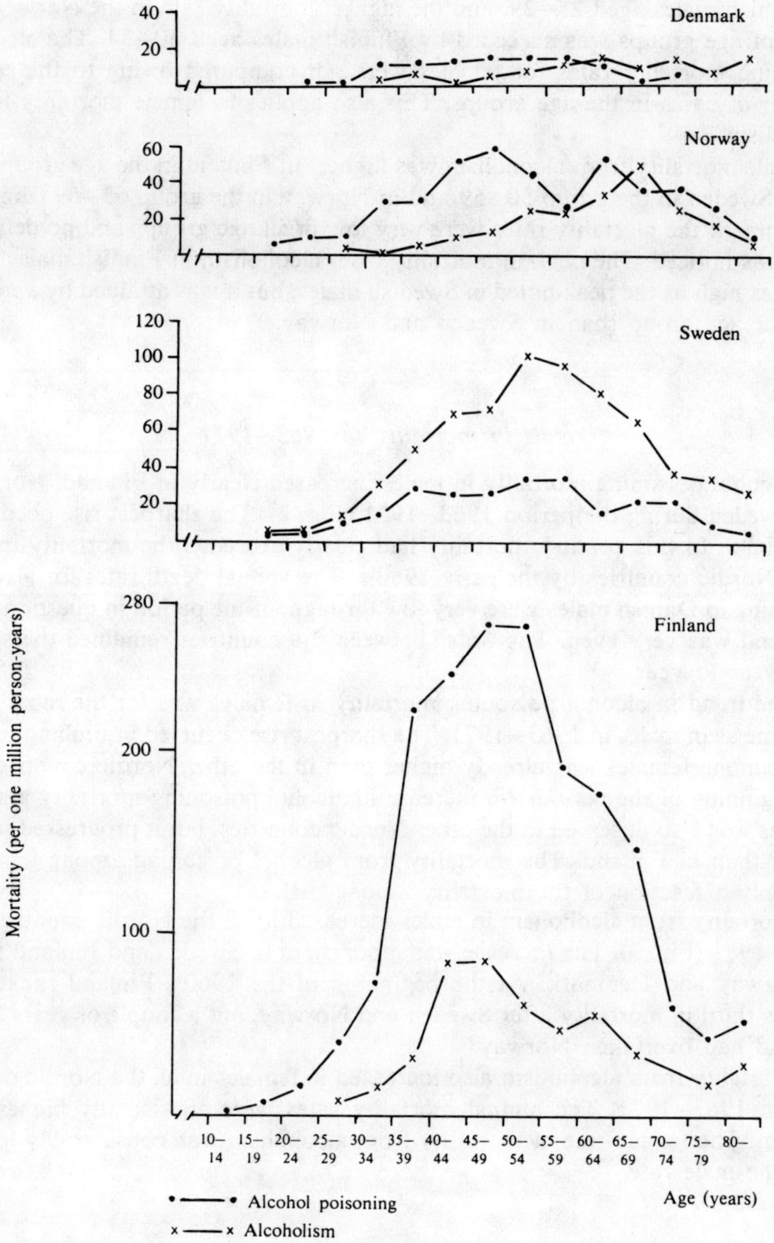

males. In the Finnish males, mortality increased sharply from the youngest to the middle-aged. The highest Swedish and Danish mortality rates were exceeded by Finnish males aged 25—29, and the highest mortality rate in the Norwegian series of age groups was exceeded by Finnish males aged 30—34. The alcohol poisoning mortality rates for females were not compared owing to the small number of cases in the age groups. This also applies to female mortality from alcoholism.

Male mortality from alcoholism was highest in Finland in the age group 40-49, in Sweden in the group 50—59 and in Norway in the group 65—69 (Fig. 1). In Denmark the mortality rates were very low in all age groups and no definite peak was noticed. The peak in mortality from alcoholism in Finnish males was about as high as the peak noted in Swedish males, but it was attained by a much younger age group than in Sweden and Norway.

Trends in mortality in 1963—1971

The alcohol poisoning mortality in males increased clearly in Finland, Norway and Sweden during the period 1963—1971 (Fig. 2). The sharpest rise occurred in Finland. In this country mortality had clearly exceeded the mortality in the other Nordic countries by the early 1960's. The annual death rates for alcohol poisoning in Danish males were very low throughout the period in question and the trend was very even. The order between the countries remained the same from year to year.

The trend in alcohol poisoning mortality in females was for the most part the same as in males in 1963—1971. The sharpest rise occurred in Finland; mortality among females was already higher than in the other Nordic countries at the beginning of the period. An increase in alcohol poisoning mortality among females was also observed in the other Nordic countries, but it progressed more slowly than in Finland. The mortality from alcohol poisoning among females was only a fraction of the mortality among males.

Mortality from alcoholism in males increased in all the Nordic countries in 1963—1971 (Fig. 3). The increase was more rapid in Sweden and Finland than in Norway and Denmark. At the beginning of the 1960's Finland ranked a narrow third in mortality after Sweden and Norway, but a couple of years later Finland had overtaken Norway.

Mortality from alcoholism also increased in females in all the Nordic countries in 1963—1971. The annual mortality rates were consistently highest in Sweden. The female rate of mortality from alcoholism was considerably lower than the male rate.

Figure 2. Trend of alcohol poisoning mortality in males in the Nordic countries 1963–1971*

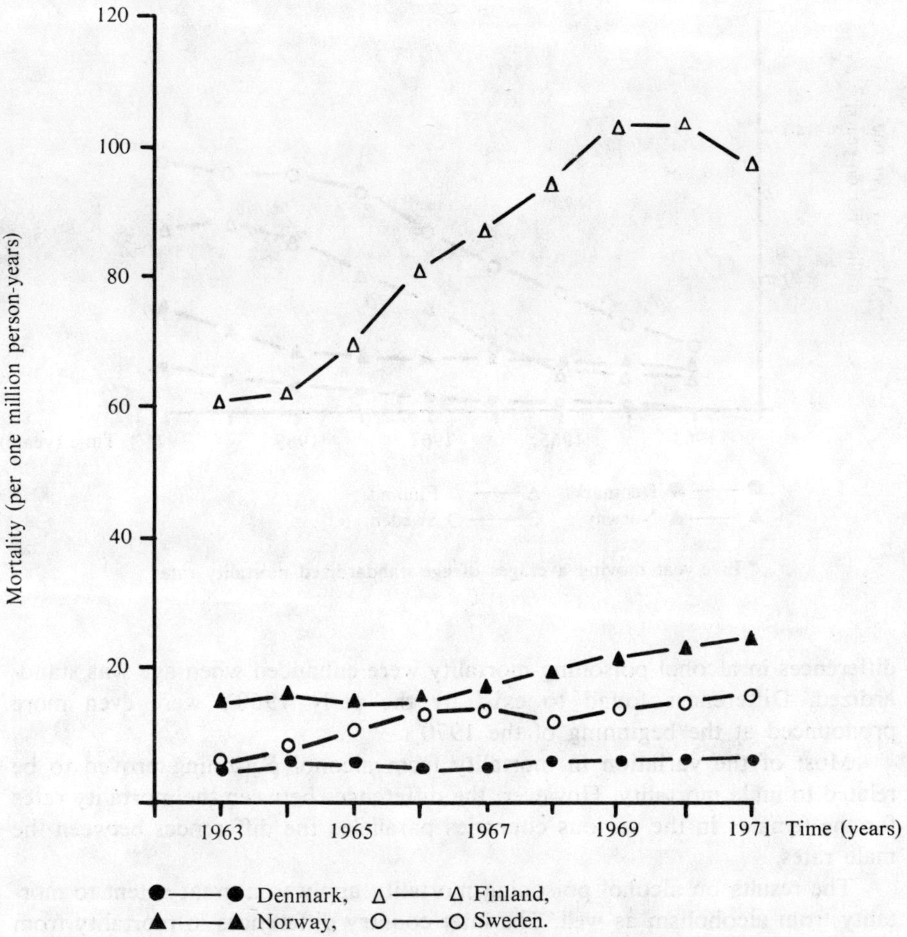

* Five-year moving averages of age-standardized mortality rates

Comment

The results obtained by analysing different aspects of alcohol poisoning mortality all confirm the view that the inter-Nordic differences in mortality are not due to chance; they are noteworthy and they must have a cause. The differences between the males in the various countries were all significant ($p < .01$). The

Figure 3. Trend of alcoholism mortality in males in the Nordic countries 1963–1971*

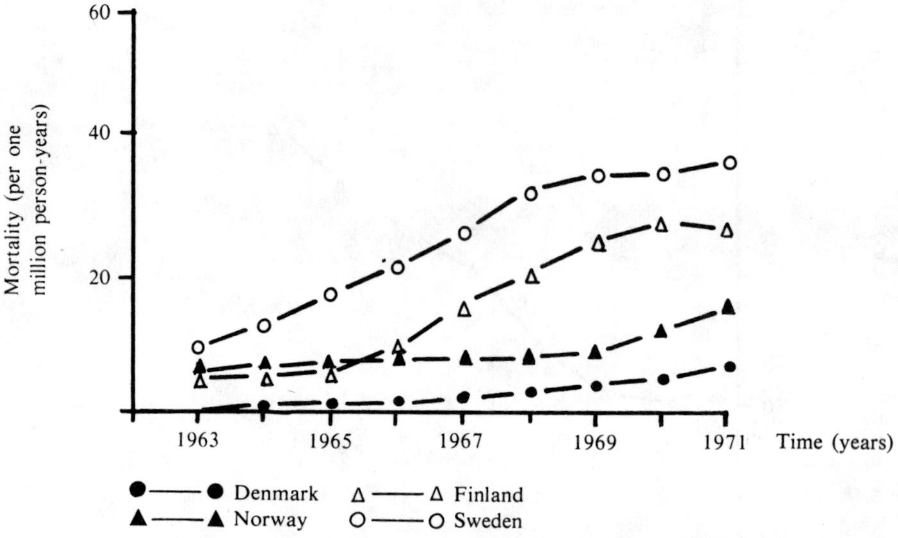

* Five-year moving averages of age-standardized mortality rates

differences in alcohol poisoning mortality were enhanced when age was standardized. Differences found to exist by the early 1960's were even more pronounced at the beginning of the 1970's.

Most of the variation in mortality from alcohol poisoning proved to be related to male mortality. However, the differences between the mortality rates for the females in the various countries paralleled the differences between the male rates.

The results on alcohol poisoning mortality apply to a great extent to mortality from alcoholism as well. The inter-country differences in mortality from alcoholism among males were all significant ($p < .01$). The annual mortality rates showed a steady upward trend during the 1963–1971 period. Age standardization did not enhance the differences; on the contrary, these were reduced. However, the age-standardized mortality rates deviated only slightly from the actual ones. As with death rates from alcohol poisoning, the proportion of female cases among the deaths from alcoholism was very small.

The most remarkable feature of the results obtained on the inter-Nordic differences in mortality from alcohol poisoning and alcoholism was that the ranking of the countries differed in the two groups. Finland occupied the first place in alcohol poisoning mortality, Sweden in mortality from alcoholism.

Mortality related to the use of alcohol has been explained mainly as a function of the average alcohol consumption of the population (Bruun et al. 1975, 15—45). Since the per capita consumption increased in all the Nordic countries in 1961—1972 (Svendsen 1976), it is tempting to attribute the rising trends in mortality from alcohol poisoning and alcoholism to the increasing alcohol consumption of the population. However, the inter-country differences, which stood out clearly during the period studied, cannot be understood only on the basis of alcohol consumption.

With regard to mortality from alcohol poisoning in 1967—1971, the ranking of the Nordic countries, in descending order, was Finland, Norway, Sweden, Denmark. The corresponding ranking for mortality from alcoholism was Sweden, Finland, Norway, Denmark. However, with regard to per capita consumption of alcohol the ranking is quite different. In 1967—1971 the consumption of 100 per cent alcohol per 15-year-old and older inhabitant in Denmark was 8.1 litres, in Sweden 6.8 litres, in Finland 5.1 litres and in Norway 4.5 litres annually (Collett 1972). On an inter-country level the correlation between alcohol consumption and mortality from alcohol poisoning and alcoholism is poor, in contrast to what has been observed for mortality from liver cirrhosis. Explanations other than the level of total alcohol consumption for the inter-country variation in mortality from alcohol poisoning and alcoholism must be looked for.

V
DISTRIBUTION BY PROVINCE OF MORTALITY FROM ALCOHOL POISONING AND ALCOHOLISM IN THE NORDIC COUNTRIES

A survey of the mortality rates for alcohol poisoning and alcoholism in different provinces may be informative with regard to the causes influencing this mortality. The consumption of alcohol is larger in urban areas than in rural districts. Lonely, isolated and rootless people who seek consolation in the bottle are more numerous in big cities. Obscure deaths are more thoroughly investigated in densely populated urban areas which have greater resources at their command. For these reasons mortality from alcohol poisoning and alcoholism might be expected to be highest in the urban areas. On the other hand, uncontrolled drinking is often encountered among isolated people living in sparsely inhabited regions. The physically hard work of some occupational groups is considered a justification for violent pleasures. A comparison of mortality by province may therefore be of assistance in assessing the weight of the different factors in the complex pattern of causes influencing mortality from alcohol poisoning and alcoholism.

Material and methods

The mortality rates for alcohol poisoning and alcoholism in the different provinces in Finland, Sweden and Norway were calculated as averages for the period 1967–1971. Denmark was excluded from comparison, since no interesting contribution to the results could be anticipated due to the small numbers of cases and the uniformly high density of population in this country. The numbers of deaths were obtained from the data base of this investigation and represent either all deaths that had occurred in the country in question or estimates based on samples. The estimates were obtained by multiplying the number of cases in a province as indicated in the sample by the ratio between all deaths and the sampled cases. The mortality rates by province are estimates with regard to mortality from alcoholism in Sweden and with regard to mortality from both alcoholism and alcohol poisoning in Finland. The population averages used for the period 1967—1971 are either means of the figures for the turn of the year 1966/67 and for the turn of the year 1971/72 or means calculated on the mid-year populations for 1967 and 1971. The differences in mortality were considered significant provided the 99 per cent confidence intervals using the Poisson distribution did not coincide.

Results

Alcohol poisoning mortality in different provinces in Finland, Norway and Sweden

The distribution of alcohol poisoning mortality by province varied greatly between the countries. In Norway mortality was concentrated in Oslo, while no clear differences were observed between any other provinces (Fig. 4). Mortality in Oslo was 35 and varied in the other parts of the country between 4 and 20 per one million person-years (Fig. 4). In Norway 35 per cent of the alcohol poisoning deaths occurred in Oslo.

In Sweden mortality from alcohol poisoning was very evenly distributed between the different provinces and the rates were low (Fig. 4). No clear differences between the different provinces were observed.

Finland was found to comprise both high-mortality and low-mortality provinces (Fig. 4). In general, mortality was clearly higher than in Norway and Sweden. In addition, a concentration of deaths was noticed in the northern parts of the country, in contrast to Norway and Sweden. Mortality was highest in the provinces of Oulu and Lapland, with figures of 79 and 75 per one million person-years. Mortality was also higher in the province of Central Finland than in the province of Uusimaa, which is the most highly industrialized part of Finland. The mortality rates for the provinces in east and west Finland were lower than the figures for north and south Finland. The mortality rate for the province of Oulu was significantly higher than the rates for the provinces of Vaasa and Häme ($p < .01$). The figures for the provinces of Lapland, Central Finland and Uusimaa were higher than the mortality rate for the province of Häme ($p < .01$).

The mortality rate for alcohol poisoning in the province of Åland was surprisingly high (Fig. 4). However, in reality this result is not attributable to a high mortality; it is due to technical circumstances related to the collection of material. The mortality rate is based on only two deaths. None of these persons was registered in Åland. They were visitors whose deaths were recorded *de facto* in this province. In the official Finnish statistics which are based on *de jure*

Figure 4. Alcohol poisoning mortality by province in Finland[1]*, Norway*[2] *and Sweden*[2]

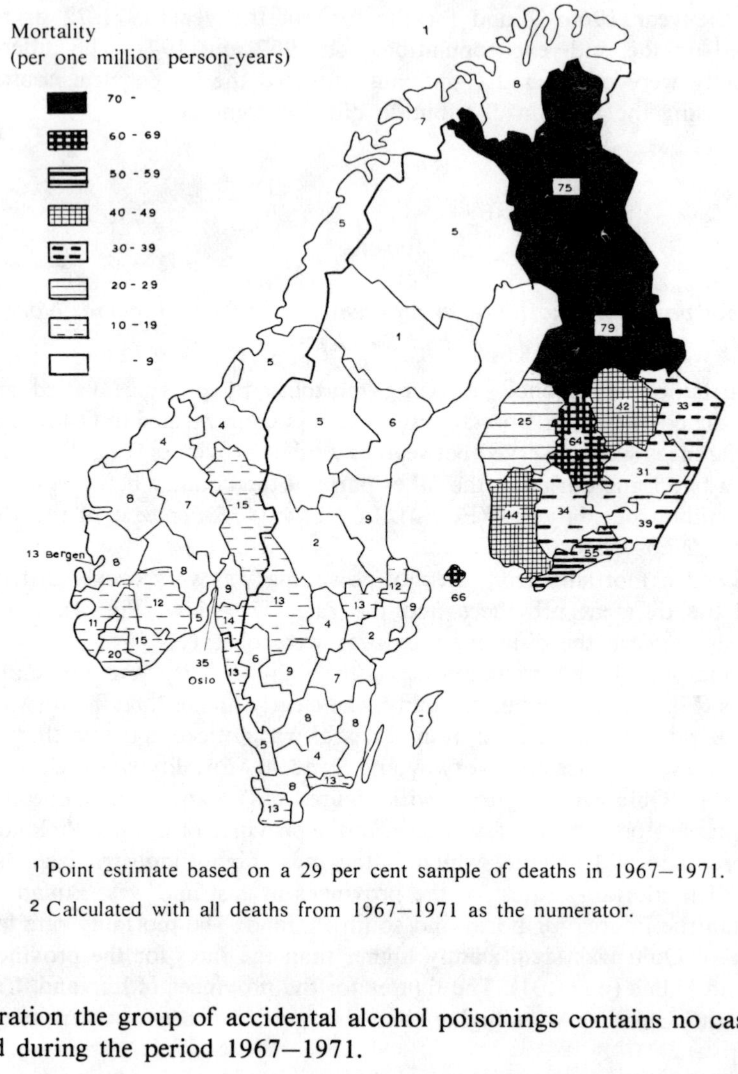

[1] Point estimate based on a 29 per cent sample of deaths in 1967–1971.
[2] Calculated with all deaths from 1967–1971 as the numerator.

registration the group of accidental alcohol poisonings contains no case from Åland during the period 1967–1971.

Mortality from alcoholism in different provinces in Finland and Sweden

In Sweden, mortality from alcoholism was greatest in the province of Stockholm, with a figure of 69 per one million person-years (Fig. 5). The mortality rate for the province of Stockholm was significantly higher than the rates

Figure 5. Alcoholism mortality by province in Finland[1] and Sweden[2]

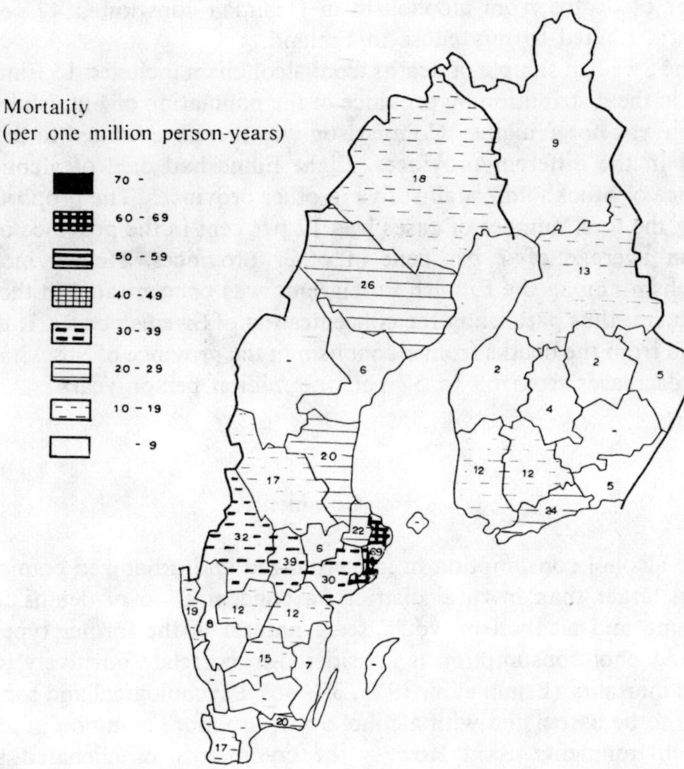

[1] Point estimate based on a 43 per cent sample of deaths in 1967–1971.
[2] Point estimate based on a 20 per cent sample of deaths in 1969–1971.

for the provinces of Östergötland, Kalmar, Malmöhus, Göteborg, Bohus, Älvsborg, Skaraborg, Västmanland, Kronoberg, Gotland, Kristianstad, Halland and Jämtland ($p < .01$). Mortality was also high in other provinces in the central part of the country (30–39 per one million person-years) compared with the rates for the provinces in the north and south (0–26 per one million person-years). In general, the differences were not significant owing to the small numbers of cases.

There was a more pronounced concentration of deaths from alcoholism in Finland than in Sweden (Fig. 5). The province of Uusimaa had the highest mortality rate, 24, against a variation from zero to 15 per one million person-years in the other provinces. The figure for Uusimaa was significantly higher than the figures for the provinces of Kuopio, Vaasa, Mikkeli and Åland ($p < .01$). The number of deaths from alcoholism in Uusimaa constituted 47 per cent of all deaths attributed to this cause in Finland.

The Swedish sample of deaths from alcoholism included 13 Finnish citizens. Data on the distribution by province of the population of Finnish immigrants in Sweden was not available. Comparison was therefore limited to the numbers of deaths in the different provinces. Eight Finns had died of alcoholism in the province of Stockholm, against five in other provinces. The proportion of Finns among the total number of cases was 17 per cent in the province of Stockholm and an average of 7 per cent in other provinces. Hence, mortality from alcoholism among the Finnish immigrants was concentrated in the province of Stockholm, thus paralleling the concentration of Swedish cases. If the Finns are omitted from the deaths from alcoholism in the province of Stockholm, the mortality decreases from 69 to 57 per one million person-years.

Comment

As the alcohol consumption in industrialized and urbanized communities is in general larger than in rural districts, a concentration of deaths from alcohol poisoning and alcoholism would seem natural in the former type of environment. Alcohol consumption is considered to correlate positively with alcohol-related mortality (Bruun et al. 1975, 30—45). Psychological and social problems known to be associated with alcohol abuse are more common in urban than in rural environments. Skid Row — the community of alienated and rootless vagrants — is a typically urban phenomenon. In cities people live and often also die alone. Quite often a police inquiry and autopsy are required to establish the cause of death, and urban authorities have relatively greater scope for ordering such inquiries. All these factors might be expected to influence the distribution of mortality by province. In part, the present results complied with this assumption. There was a noticeable concentration of deaths from alcohol poisoning in Oslo in Norway, and from alcoholism in the province of Stockholm in Sweden and the province of Uusimaa in Finland. However, the variation in alcohol poisoning mortality in Finland cannot be explained in the same way.

It has been reported that uncontrolled use of alcohol lasts for days not only among chronic alcoholics, but also at times among the population of the sparsely inhabited northern regions. In the countryside in northern Norway alcohol is on average used very sparingly, but on great holidays groups of men sound asleep after a good booze-up may be found obstructing the public highways (Irgens-Jensen 1965, 30—31). In an interview-study carried out in Finnish Lapland the cassier of a logging camp (Sariola 1956, 61) gave the following account of the logger's daily experience of isolation and hard work, which eventually explodes in a craving for Dionysian revels:

"After the *jätkä* has toiled for a month or two and slaved, without any variety or recreation, slept badly in unsatisfactory cabins, and got to be thoroughly bitter, he'll have to go to Rovaniemi. He'll get mentally loaded, in these conditions, to such an extent that the desire for variety will be fed unwisely, by drinking heavily as long as there is some cash left in the pockets. He'll swallow in senselessly. Here, the *jätkä's* nerves get irritated. The moment he is in Rovaniemi, he'll start for the liquor store or for the bootlegger, and he'll satisfy his desire for recreation and change in a primitive and uncontrolled manner. He takes his fun as seriously as his work, and he wants to get a quick satisfaction."

Violent drinking thus occurs in sparsely inhabited provinces also, but how does it influence alcohol poisoning mortality? In this respect the Nordic countries seem to differ clearly from each other. In Norway and Sweden mortality is low in the northern provinces, while the opposite is the case in Finland. The highest mortality rates were noted in the sparsely populated provinces of Oulu, Lapland and Central Finland. The most industrialized province, that of Uusimaa, ranks after these three in mortality. The impression is given that uncontrolled drinking is so much more typical of the Finns that this factor is reflected in a high mortality even in provinces with a low alcohol consumption.

The higher alcohol poisoning mortality in the sparsely populated Finnish provinces compared with corresponding regions in Norway and Sweden may in part be due to the fact that obscure deaths are more often subjected to postmortem examination in Finland, owing to effective organization on the province level of the medicolegal system of cause-of-death inquiries. However, evidence of a relatively frequent occurrence of alcohol-related health problems in the northern and eastern parts of Finland has also been presented in previous investigations. On the basis of mortality from liver cirrhosis, the prevalence of alcoholism has been estimated as being rather high in central and east Finland (Kerosuo 1970). The frequency of occupational disability attributed to alcoholism was higher in the rural districts of northern and eastern Finland than in the rural districts of southern and western Finland (Poikolainen et al. 1973). The strikingly low alcohol poisoning mortality in the province of Åland, the archipelago which belongs to Finland although it is mainly inhabited by a Swedish-speaking population, also suggests that cultural differences in drinking habits are of importance.

During the period covered by this study, 1967–1971, none of the resident population of Åland died of alcohol poisoning, although this was the fate of two visitors. A survey of the alcohol poisoning mortality statistics for 1930–1949 revealed one death, which was clearly due to accidental ingestion of methanol, while 929 persons died of alcohol poisoning in other parts of Finland during the same period (Huhtala 1951).

VI
CAUSE-OF-DEATH INQUIRIES AND ALCOHOL POISONING MORTALITY

In the investigation of inter-country variations in alcohol poisoning mortality, attention must be paid to the different systems used to ascertain the causes of death. The thoroughness of cause-of-death inquiries may influence the reliability of the diagnoses made. It may be difficult to certify that alcohol poisoning was the cause of death unless careful examinations are performed. Diagnostic reliability is enhanced if no other cause of death was demonstrable.

The inference that the thoroughness of cause-of-death inquiries affects the number of diagnoses of deaths from alcohol poisoning in the Nordic countries can be made on two conditions. First, it must be shown that these countries differ from each other in the degree of thoroughness and, second, that greater thoroughness increases the number of diagnoses.

Thoroughness of cause-of-death inquiries in the Nordic countries

In this study, the expression thoroughness of cause-of-death inquiries is used for the total amount of information by which the causes of death are identified. In the individual case, the degree of thoroughness depends on the number and quality of the examinations performed. Autopsy occupies a key position, as autopsy determines whether chemical, histological and other examinations be performed. The proportion of autopsied cases may therefore be used as a crude indicator of the degree of thoroughness.

The various Nordic countries differed widely in the ratio of autopsied cases to the total number of deaths in 1967–1971. Autopsy was performed in Denmark and Sweden in about half the cases, in Finland in about one-third and in Norway in about one-tenth (Table 10). However, the frequency of medicolegal autopsies is of particular interest in a study on mortality from alcohol poisoning, since a large proportion of these deaths are sudden and occur outside hospitals for no apparent reason. Hence, they are likely to be subject to medicolegal examination. The frequency of medicolegal autopsies in

Table 10. Ratio of autopsied cases to all deaths in the Nordic countries

	Denmark Per cent	Finland Per cent	Norway Per cent	Sweden Per cent
Medicolegal autopsies[1]	2	13	1[e]	7
All autopsies[1]	44	31	12	47
Autopsies among victims of accidents, poisoning and violence[2]	33	69	12	57

[1]Average for 1967–1971.
[2]ICD class XVII (Seventh Revision). Average for 1966–1968. Source: Bolander 1971, 30.

1967–1971 was clearly greater in Finland (13 per cent) than in Sweden (7 per cent) and Denmark (2 per cent). No exact information was obtained from Norway, but on the basis of data for the years 1966–1969 (Oikeuslääketieteellisten... 1971, 24) the ratio of medicolegally autopsied deaths to all deaths was estimated at about one per cent.

The thoroughness in inquiring into alcohol poisoning deaths may also be assessed by determining the proportion of autopsies carried out on those whose death was recorded as caused by accidents, poisoning and violence. In 1966–1968 the autopsy ratio in this ICD category was clearly highest in Finland (Table 10). The conclusion may be ventured that the degree of thoroughness in inquiring into deaths attributed to alcohol poisoning was greatest in Finland. Judging by the same criterion, Sweden ranked second, Denmark third and Norway fourth. The differences between the countries demanded a closer study of the significance of cause-of-death inquiries.

Organization of medicolegal cause-of-death inquiries in the Nordic countries

The statutes relating to medicolegal inquiries into the causes of deaths and the activities of the medicolegal organizations in the different Nordic countries were compared in order to clarify the effect of the thoroughness of cause-of-death inquiries on the alcohol poisoning mortality rates. The next section deals with the principal similarities and differences between the various Nordic organizations. A more detailed account is given in Appendix 1. The comparison relates to the organization and function of the medicolegal services in 1967–1971.*

* The Finnish medicolegal services have been modified by a new law on the examination of the cause of death (1. 6. 1973/459) in 1974.

Statutes

In all the Nordic countries the decision that a medicolegal investigation be performed is taken by the police. In contrast, the statutes stating when the police should be notified about a death and in what circumstances the police should find it necessary to inquire into the cause of death vary with the country.

Deaths should first be notified either to the police or to a physician. The statutes stating what cases physicians ought to report to the police as suspicious vary in the Nordic countries. In Finland and Sweden, a physician is in duty bound to notify the police about all cases in which foul play, injury or poisoning may be suspected or the cause of death cannot be definitely established. The National Board of Health has advised Finnish physicians not to issue a death certificate if there are any grounds for suspecting that an accident, foul play or poisoning is involved, or if death has been sudden or violent and no obvious cause can be established (Isotalo 1970, 132). In Denmark, physicians are duty bound to notify the police only about cases in which foul play may be suspected or suicide or an accident is the cause of death (Gormsen 1973, 82). In Norway, a physician is not obliged to report a case to the police even if he or she is reluctant to sign a death certificate stating that there are no grounds for suspecting foul play. Norwegian physicians are in duty bound to notify the police only about deaths as stipulated in § 263 of the Act of 1887 on the procedure in criminal cases. This originally only affected relatives of the deceased; hence, the duty of notification mainly applies to cases in which relatives may be suspected of criminal involvement (Lundevall 1973, 45–46).

When notified about an obscure death, the police decide on the desirability for an autopsy or other examinations designed to clarify the cause of death, as stipulated in the statutes. In all the Nordic countries the police are obliged to order a medicolegal investigation if there are any grounds for suspecting foul play. This is clearly stated in the laws and statutes. With regard to inquiries into other cases the statutes are less definite.

The Danish police are not duty bound to order a medicolegal autopsy unless foul play is suspected or known to be linked in some way with the death. In obscure cases in which it is deemed desirable to clarify the cause of death the police may ask for what is called a police autopsy (Gormsen 1973, 101–102). However, if the case is not considered interesting, the police may desist from ordering a medicolegal autopsy (Gormsen 1973, 122).

There is some ambiguity in the Finnish statutes as to when the police should order a medicolegal autopsy; they are authorized to consider this possibility in all cases in which the cause of death cannot otherwise be established with certainty. The interpretation of the statutes has been a matter of some debate. In general, the medical profession has been of the opinion that all unexpected deaths and deaths caused by accident, suicide or poisoning should be subject to autopsy, whereas the police have considered autopsy to be necessary only where crime was suspected (Oikeuslääketieteellisten... 1971, 74–75).

In Norway, the police have the right to determine when a death is considered to be connected with foul play and in such cases to order an autopsy (Lundevall 1973, 21). Otherwise the police are not obliged to interfere.

The Swedish police use their own discretion with regard to whether an autopsy should be carried out. The police are informed as to the desirability of autopsy by the physician who has examined the deceased and then decide in the matter as they think fit. The physician is authorized to require of the police a more thorough investigation if this is deemed necessary (Socialstyrelsen 1971). The statutes are set out in general terms and are elastic.

In connection with obscure deaths a situation may arise in which the physician regards supplementary examinations as necessary and the police disagree. The decision may then depend on the physician's obligation to issue a death certificate without the evidence obtained from such examinations. The obligation to write a death certificate differs with the country. Finnish physicians are forbidden to issue a death certificate before a police inquiry has been carried out unless the deceased was under medical care during his or her last illness or if there is a suspicion of accident, crime or poisoning (Isotalo 1970, 132). As with their Finnish colleagues, Swedish physicians have the right to refuse to write a death certificate if they find that the examination of the deceased warrants further examinations. Danish physicians, on the other hand, are obliged to issue a death certificate even without the evidence of supplementary examinations, if such examinations are deemed unnecessary by the police (Gormsen 1973, 82). A Norwegian physician who has inspected the dead body is obliged to write a death certificate. If no other physician can be called, a medical officer inspects the body. Physicians may refuse to sign a statement to the effect that there are no grounds for suspicion of foul play, but this does not mean that the police must be notified about the case.

Structure

At the time of this investigation autopsy units were clearly more numerous in Finland than in the other Nordic countries. Autopsies were performed by physicians in 12 provinces and at the departments of forensic medicine in Helsinki, Turku and Oulu. Hence, the number of autopsy units in operation was 15. In Sweden, these activities were centralized so that autopsies were performed at five national institutes of forensic medicine. In Denmark, medicolegal autopsies were performed at three university institutes of forensic medicine. Norway had two such institutes, but medicolegal autopsies were also carried out at the departments of pathology of the largest hospitals.

Activity

The medicolegal autopsy ratios were calculated on all deaths recorded in the official statistics in the Nordic countries during the period 1967–1971. A marked and continuous increase in the medicolegal autopsy ratio was noticed in Finland and Sweden. Finland had the highest ratio, 14.9 per cent in 1971, and the increase of this ratio from 1967 was 30 per cent. In Sweden the autopsy ratio was 9.9 per cent in 1971, and the increase from 1967 was as much as 74 per cent.

In Denmark no notable change in the frequency of medicolegal autopsies was observed, but the ratio of medicolegal external inspections, which was remarkably high in Denmark compared with the other Nordic countries – 9.6 per cent in 1971 – increased by 13 per cent.

No information on the frequency of medicolegal autopsies was obtained from Norway, but data on all autopsies performed during the study period was available. The autopsy ratio, calculated on all deaths, did not change to any notable degree. It may be assumed that no appreciable change occurred in the frequency of medicolegal autopsies, either.

As regards blood ethanol determinations performed post mortem, data suitable for purposes of comparison was not available. Adequate information was only obtained from Denmark, where the ethanol concentration had been determined in almost 3 per cent of all deaths. The corresponding figure for Finland may be estimated at about 3–4 per cent on the basis of the data obtained over a period of two years. No precise data was forthcoming from Sweden and Norway, but it is known that various chemical examinations were performed in 1972 in Sweden in about 4 per cent of all deaths and that over four analyses were performed in each case examined. It may therefore be assumed that the frequency of postmortal blood ethanol determinations was about the same in Sweden as in Denmark and Finland.

Comment

The activities of the organizations which conduct medicolegal cause-of-death inquiries were found to be compatible with the statutes regulating them. The statutes constitute the framework setting the limits for these activities. In Finland and Sweden the statutes allow thorough inquiries into deaths suspected to be caused by poisoning, whereas the task of the medicolegal organizations in Denmark and Norway is concerned with the disclosure of crimes. The effect of limiting the aims of cause-of-death inquiries in these countries is observable at all points that were subject to analysis.

In Norway the possibilities for investigating deaths not suspected to be caused by foul play are fewer than in Denmark. Although the Danish, like the Norwegian, statutes are mainly concerned with the clarification of crimes, the former permit "police autopsies" even if no crime is thought to be involved. Moreover, a chemical examination is often performed in Denmark in connection with medicolegal external inspection of the dead body. The frequency of postmortal blood alcohol determinations calculated on all deaths in Denmark was almost as high as in Finland, despite the great difference in the autopsy ratio.

The legislative restriction of the Danish and Norwegian medicolegal autopsy systems as instruments for the clarification of crimes explains why the autopsy ratios in these countries remained small throughout the period 1967–1971, while the autopsy ratios in Sweden and Finland increased to a marked degree. The small number of autopsies together with the limitations imposed on the medicolegal services mean that deaths by poisoning, which are thoroughly investigated in Sweden and Finland, are likely in some instances to be studied only superficially in Denmark and Norway. This assumption applies in particular to Norway, where the autopsy ratio was lowest and the scope of cause-of-death inquiries most restricted by the statutes.

Association between the thoroughness of cause-of-death inquiries and poisoning mortality

By a simple process of reasoning it may be assumed that the thoroughness of cause-of-death inquiries influences the mortality rate for a certain cause of death when this cause is not obvious. If no examinations are performed, no reliable diagnoses will be made. On the other hand, if all deaths are examined by all available means, it may be assumed that all deaths from the cause in question which can be diagnosed by current techniques and on the basis of present-day knowledge will be detected. Some kind of association may thus be presumed to exist between the thoroughness of cause-of-death inquiries and the number of diagnosed cases. However, it is not sufficient that an association may be presumed to exist; the point at issue is the kind and strength of the association. In the following sections this point will be analysed on the basis of empirical data.

Material and methods

An evaluation of the association between alcohol poisoning mortality and the thoroughness of cause-of-death inquiries presupposes (1) that other factors influencing the mortality are standardized, (2) that an appropriate observation unit is found and (3) that an appropriate data base is available. In the Nordic countries, these criteria are satisfactorily fulfilled only by the Finnish data.

The variation of the other factors influencing alcohol poisoning mortality may be reduced by analysing the material on an intra-country basis. Thus, although crudely restricted, some of the variation still remains. However, the large differences in mortality between the Nordic countries seem to indicate that most of the variation is inter-country. Evaluation by country is thus an appropriate approach.

The nature of the problem presupposes that a geographical area is used as the observation unit. In the Nordic countries, a province is an appropriate unit. As the majority of fatal alcohol poisonings consist of sudden deaths occurring outside hospitals, they are likely to be subjected to medicolegal cause-of-death inquiries. It is therefore an advantage if the medicolegal services are organized on a province basis and if cause-of-death inquiries are carried out within the framework of this organization, as they are in Finland.

Medicolegal autopsies belong in Finland to the duties of the provincial medical officers. The university departments of forensic medicine are also mainly concerned with autopsies of deaths that have occurred within the province in which the university is located. Medicolegal cause-of-death inquiries are more frequently carried out in Finland than in the other Nordic countries (Table 10). This applies in particular to cases of poisoning. The ratio of medicolegal autopsies to all alcohol poisoning deaths was 97 per cent in Finland, 59 per cent in Denmark, 48 per cent in Norway and 75 per cent in Sweden during the study period (Table 11). The fact that no medical autopsies were performed in Finland on subjects who had died of alcohol poisoning, in contrast to Sweden and Norway, and that no medicolegal external inspections were made, as in Denmark, justifies the use of the medicolegal autopsy ratio as an indicator of the thoroughness of cause-of-death inquiries with regard to alcohol poisoning deaths in Finland, particularly when one considers that almost all of those who died of alcohol poisoning were medicolegally examined in this country. Moreover, it was not possible in Finland to conduct any forensic chemical analysis necessary for the demonstration of blood alcohol except in connection

Table 11. Ratio of autopsied cases to all deaths from alcohol poisoning or alcoholism by type of autopsy in the study groups

	Alcohol poisoning				Alcoholism	
Type of autopsy	Denmark Per cent	Finland Per cent	Norway Per cent	Sweden [a] Per cent	Finland Per cent	Sweden [a] Per cent
Medicolegal autopsy	59	97	48	75	73	63
Medical autopsy	–	–	15	14	–	20
Number of deaths	106	328	238	325	118	115

with medicolegal cause-of-death inquiries (Oikeuslääketieteellisten... 1971, 90–91), and almost all medicolegal cause-of-death inquiries (98.5 per cent of those carried out in 1967–1971) implied autopsy.

In Finland, information on the numbers of medicolegal autopsies performed in the different provinces is obtainable from the official cause-of-death statistics. Alcohol poisoning mortality rates by province have not been tabulated, but the official statistics give the numbers of accidental poisoning deaths that have occurred in the different provinces. Accidental poisoning deaths may well be used in the analysis instead of alcohol poisoning deaths, because a large proportion of the accidental deaths by poisoning are alcohol poisoning deaths (69 per cent during the period 1963–1971) and alcohol poisoning deaths and other deaths by poisoning are closely related diagnostic problems.

It was decided to compare the frequency of medicolegal autopsies with the frequency of accidental poisoning deaths by province in Finland. Data was collected over as many years as possible in order to acquire a sufficient number of observations. The first year for which medicolegal and clinical autopsies had been separately recorded in the statistics was 1963, and the last year for which all the required data was obtained was 1971. The chronological series comprised nine years, and as there are 12 provinces in Finland, the number of observations was 108.

As the object of analysis was the connection between the frequency of accidental deaths by poisoning and the frequency of medicolegal autopsies, it was considered appropriate to use the proportion of accidental poisonings among all deaths to represent the frequency instead of the mortality rate.

Results

The medicolegal autopsy ratios varied from 1.9 to 23.2 per cent, and the frequency of accidental poisonings varied from 0 to 13.4 per mille. There was a conspicuous covariation between the variables (Fig. 6). The product-moment correlation coefficient between the variables was + .48. The coefficient differed very significantly from zero ($p < .001$, two sided *t*-test).

As the province of Åland is exceptional in its small number of alcohol poisoning deaths (p. 61), and as it was assumed that the drinking habits in this area may differ from the drinking habits in other parts of the country, the correlation between the variables was also calculated after omission of the figures for Åland. Thus calculated, the correlation coefficient was + .43 ($p < .001$, two-sided *t*-test). Thus, the omission of Åland does not notably influence the covariation.

The correlation between the medicolegal autopsy ratios and the frequency of poisoning deaths is so strong that it clearly proves the existence of a covariation. According to variance interpretation of the correlation coefficient the

Figure 6. Ratio of accidental fatal poisonings and ratio of medicolegal autopsies to all deaths in Finnish provinces 1963–1971

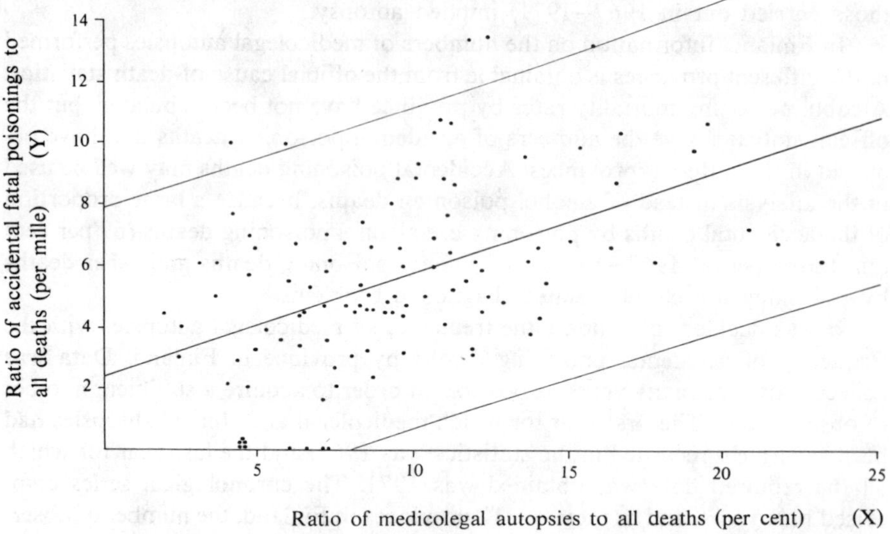

The regression function (± half of the 95 per cent tolerance intervals) of Y on X, estimated by the method of the sum of least squares, is $Y = 0.33\ X + 2.45\ (\pm \sqrt{27.305 + 0.011\ (X-9.506)^2})$.

variation of the autopsy ratios explains 23 per cent of the variation in the frequency of poisoning deaths in the total material and 19 per cent if Åland is omitted.

When analysing the connection between the medicolegal autopsy ratios and the frequency of poisoning deaths by province over nine consecutive years, a positive correlation between the variables was observed in most provinces. A particularly clear covariation suggesting a positive linear correlation was observed in those provinces in which the alcohol poisoning mortality was high, i.e. the provinces of Central Finland, Oulu and Lapland. A positive correlation also seemed to exist in the provinces of Turku and Pori, Kuopio, Mikkeli, North Karelia and Kymi. By contrast, no clear correlation was noted for the provinces of Häme and Vaasa, and in Uusimaa the correlation seemed to be negative.

The linear regression of the ratio of accidental deaths by poisoning to all deaths (Y) on the ratio of medicolegal autopsies to all deaths (X), estimated by the method of the sum of least squares, was $Y = 0.33\ X + 2.45$. The linear model predicts the change in the frequency of poisoning deaths associated with a change in the autopsy ratio. The 95 per cent confidence limits of the regression coefficient were 0.18—0.48 and the tolerance intervals for Y under the condition X were also wide (Fig. 6, for computation see Diem and Lentner 1973, 177). The accuracy of prediction of the number of fatal poisonings from the number of autopsies was, therefore, poor.

Comment

A clear positive correlation was observed between the medicolegal autopsy ratios and the frequencies of accidental deaths by poisoning. The correlation coefficients implied that the variation in the frequency of medicolegal autopsies explained about one-fifth of the variation in poisoning mortality.

About four-fifths of the variation in the frequency of poisoning deaths remained unexplained. This variation may be attributed to other factors influencing the frequency of fatal alcohol poisonings, such as drinking habits and differences in diagnostic practice and factors influencing the mortality from other kinds of accidental poisoning.

The medicolegal autopsy ratios varied in the material from 1.9 to 23.2 per cent. The range of variation corresponds fairly well to the variation existing on an inter-country level and includes the autopsy ratios considered optimal. The appropriate frequency of medicolegal autopsies has been estimated at about 20—25 per cent, and in the 1950's the frequency varied between .01 and 26.8 per cent in different countries (Oikeuslääketieteellisten... 1971, 22). The same kind of connection as was observed in this study may also exist in other countries. Considering the shape of the connection, it might be assumed that it is limited by a ceiling, implying that the connection disappears if the frequency of medicolegal autopsies increases to a certain level. It seems possible that an increase in the frequency of medicolegal autopsies no longer raises the number of diagnosed poisoning cases to any appreciable degree, if a certain proportion of deaths occurring outside hospitals are medicolegally investigated. This ceiling perhaps lies in the area of the recommended autopsy ratio of 20—25 per cent.

It may be assumed that a connection exists only if practically all alcohol poisoning deaths are diagnosed by medicolegal autopsy. If a great many deaths from alcohol poisoning are subjected to clinical autopsy at hospitals, these autopsies must be included in an evaluation of the connection . Generalization on an inter-country level is weakened by the fact that in some countries (e.g. Denmark) deaths from alcohol poisoning are often diagnosed on the basis of external inspection and determination of the postmortal blood alcohol concentration. When other causes of death have not been excluded by means of autopsy, the group may include a number of cases erroneously labelled alcohol poisoning. A prerequisite for inter-country generalizations is an appropriate indicator of the thoroughness of cause-of-death inquiries.

The model expressing the connection may theoretically be used for prediction of the change in the number of alcohol poisoning deaths following upon a change in the thoroughness of cause-of-death inquiries. However, the regression equation calculated on the basis of the empirical material is not suited for this purpose, because the accuracy of the predictions is rather poor owing to the wide confidence limits of the regression coefficient and wide tolerance intervals. For this reason it was not considered appropriate to calculate estimates of mortality, standardized by means of the linear model with regard to autopsy ratios.

Since (1) a positive correlation was observed between the frequency of medicolegal autopsies and the frequency of established poisoning deaths and (2) the autopsy ratios varied considerably between the Nordic countries and (3) the statutes regulating cause-of-death inquiries restrict the scope for investigating suspected cases of poisoning more in some countries than in others, differing degrees of thoroughness of cause-of-death inquiries is one cause of the differences in alcohol poisoning mortality between the Nordic countries. Nonetheless, the positive correlation observed may be due partly not only to a real increase in the frequency of established poisoning deaths associated with an increase in the autopsy ratio, but also to an increased need for autopsies associated with an increase in the number of suspected cases of alcohol poisoning. This mechanism may in part explain the positive correlation in a chronological series, although the need for medicolegal autopsies evidently depends chiefly on factors other than the number of alcohol poisoning deaths. More confident causal conclusions would presuppose a chronological series in which medicolegal autopsies also decrease in frequency, and during the period covered by this study no such decrease occurred.

The thoroughness of medicolegal cause-of-death inquiries seems to influence the number of established alcohol poisoning deaths. However, the effect of the thoroughness cannot be considered as causally unquestionable, and the effect on the differences in mortality cannot be measured exactly.

VII
DIAGNOSTIC DIFFERENCES

Differences between Finland and Sweden in mortality from alcohol poisoning and alcoholism

It was assumed from the official mortality rates for alcohol poisoning and alcoholism that a proportion of cases which in Finland would be labelled alcohol poisoning deaths, are considered in Sweden to be caused by alcoholism. This assumption was tested by comparing the characteristics of alcohol poisoning deaths and deaths attributed to alcoholism in Finland and Sweden.

Methods

The possible presence of diagnostic differences was evaluated by means of five alcohol-related variables. Of these, fatty liver and pancreatitis may be results of heavy drinking. A Skid Row way of life and the consumption of industrial alcohols provide evidence of a social decline following upon a long-standing heavy use of alcohol. The postmortal blood ethanol concentration is related to drinking immediately prior to death and reflects the acute and lethal effects of alcohol.

The assumption that these variables are of essential importance constituted the basis for the tests for diagnostic differences. If deaths from alcohol poisoning and from alcoholism are distinguished as separate diagnostic groups, it was presumed that the two groups must differ with regard to these variables. On the other hand, if the two diagnoses are used interchangeably, the variables cannot distinguish between the two groups.

In this analysis only males were considered, so that the sex-related variation could be disregarded. The inter-country differences in alcohol poisoning mortality are, for the most part, differences in the mortality of males (Chapter 4).

The correlations between the variables compared have been expressed as relative coefficients of contingency. The relative coefficient of contingency is the ratio of the coefficient of contingency (Spiegel 1961, 204) to the theoretical maximum value for this coefficient.

In Finland, the group of deaths from alcohol poisoning and that of deaths from alcoholism clearly differed from each other with regard to the alcohol-related factors for which they were tested; in Sweden this was not the case (Table 12). In Finland fatty liver and pancreatitis were far more common in the alcoholism group than in the alcohol poisoning group. The proportion of Skid Row alcoholics was also markedly larger in the former group, whereas the proportion of subjects who had ingested industrial alcohol was larger in the latter group than among those who had died of alcoholism, but the difference and the number of cases on which it was calculated were small.

There was also, in Finland, a clear difference in postmortal blood ethanol concentration between the two diagnostic groups. The mean ethanol concentration was over 1.5 per mille higher in the alcohol poisoning group than in the group of deaths from alcoholism (Table 12). The shape of the distributions of the ethanol concentration showed that the two groups were clearly different, as only a fraction of the alcohol poisoning cases fell within the area of distribution of the alcoholism group and vice versa (Fig. 7).

In Sweden, no clear differences between the group of deaths from alcohol poisoning and that of deaths from alcoholism were observed with regard to the frequency of fatty liver, pancreatitis, Skid Row alcoholism or the use of industrial alcohols (Table 12), and the mean blood ethanol concentration was only 0.3 per mille higher in the alcohol poisoning group than in the alcoholism group. The distributions of the ethanol concentration were quite similar in shape (Fig. 8).

The relative coefficients of contingency measure the strength of the correlation between the frequency of alcohol-related pathological findings and the diagnostic differentiation of alcohol poisoning and alcoholism in Sweden and Finland. The coefficients were larger for Finland than for Sweden, except for the frequency of pancreatitis; on this point the difference between the two countries was small (Table 13). Moreover, the associations between the diagnostic dichotomy and the frequency of the various findings were all more significant in Finland ($p = .067 - .000$) than in Sweden ($p = .745 - .096$). Thus, it appears that the variables tested clearly distinguish alcohol poisoning deaths from deaths caused by alcoholism in Finland, but not in Sweden.

The similarity of the Swedish groups of alcohol poisoning deaths and deaths from alcoholism suggested that these causes of death are used interchangeably in the classification of cases. As both groups were large, the question presented itself as to where the one and where the other diagnosis is used. In order to clarify this point, the cases were tabulated by diagnostic group and by signer or origin of the death certificate (Table 14). Almost half of the diagnoses of alcoholism had been made at the National Institute of Forensic Medicine in

Table 12. Differences in alcohol-related factors between males who died of alcohol poisoning and males who died of alcoholism in Finland and Sweden

Factors	Finland		Sweden [a]	
	Alcohol poisoning	Alcoholism	Alcohol poisoning	Alcoholism
Skid Row alcoholism (per cent of cases)	40	60	14	12
Industrial alcohols found on chemical examination (per cent of cases)	17	12	12	8
Fatty liver (per cent of cases)	42	86	53	55
Pancreatitis (per cent of cases)	5	12	2	6
Post-mortem blood ethanol concentration, mean (per mille)	3.24	1.72	2.68	2.38

Table 13. Association between diagnostic classification and alcohol-related factors in Finnish and Swedish males who died of alcohol poisoning or alcoholism

Factors	Association between diagnostic classification and alcohol-related factors			
	Finland		Sweden [a]	
	C*	p-value	C*	p-value
Proportion of Skid Row alcoholics (1 df)	0.27	.002	0.16	.096
Proportion of users of industrial alcohols (1 df)	0.13	.067	0.09	.211
Proportion of fatty liver cases (1 df)	0.49	.000	0.02	.745
Proportion of pancreatitis cases (1 df)	0.18	.013	0.21	x
Post-mortem blood ethanol concentration (2 df)	0.85	.000	0.18	.111

* C = relative coefficient of contingency
Chi-square contingency test

Stockholm, whereas only about one-tenth of all alcohol poisoning deaths had been certified at this institute. The medicolegal experts working in Stockholm thus favour a diagnosis of alcoholism, while alcohol poisoning is preferred as a diagnosis at other institutes of forensic medicine.

It must also be taken into account that when a case is statistically recorded, an underlying cause of death may be codified other than that indicated on the death certificate. In connection with the collection of material, an opportunity arose in Sweden to study a group of cases, considered by the medicolegal experts as alcohol poisonings, though not statistically recorded under this code.

Figure 7. Post-mortem blood ethanol concentration among males who died of alcohol poisoning or alcoholism in Finland

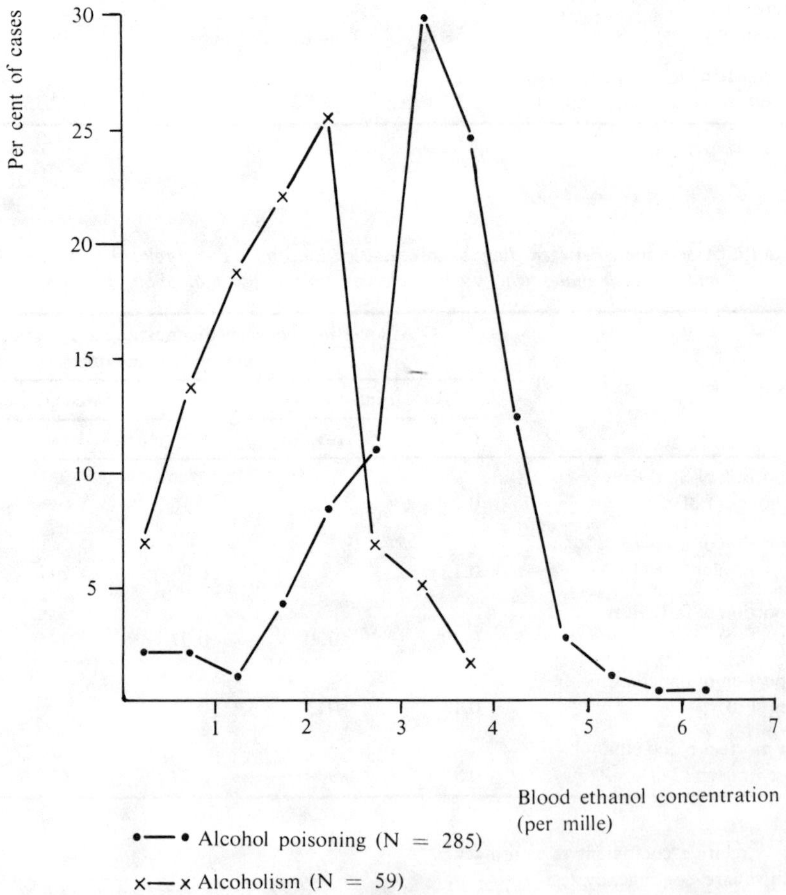

Figure 8. Post-mortem blood ethanol concentration among males who died of alcohol poisoning or alcoholism in Sweden[5]

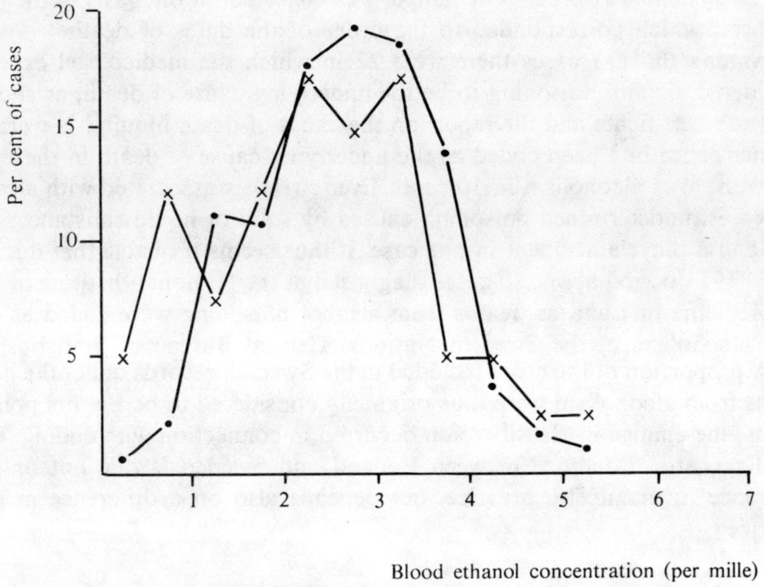

Table 14. Signers or origin of the death certificates of Swedish subjects who died of alcohol poisoning or alcoholism

Signer or origin of death certificate	Alcohol poisoning Number of cases	Alcoholism Number of cases
Medicolegal expert		
Stockholm	32	54
Uppsala	48	6
Lund	85	6
Göteborg	69	8
Umeå	9	4
Hospital physician	46	20
Certificate obtained from abroad	7	–
Certificate not found	3	–
Total	325	115

From the archives of the National Institute of Forensic Medicine in Lund, cases were collected in which alcohol had been demonstrated post mortem. The total number of such cases examined at this institute in 1967—1971 was 234. From these, a systematic 50 per cent sample was collected on the basis of the journal numbers, which corresponded to the order of the dates of death.

Among the 117 cases there were 22 in which the medicolegal expert had considered alcohol poisoning to be the underlying cause of death, as shown by the death certificate and the report on the cause-of-death inquiry. Nevertheless, another cause had been coded as the underlying cause of death in these cases. The cause was alcoholism in 10 cases, liver cirrhosis associated with alcohol in two cases, undetermined poisoning caused by solid or liquid substances in one case and a bicycle accident in one case. It thus seems probable that during the 1967—1971 period about 20 cases diagnosed at the National Institute of Forensic Medicine in Lund as deaths from alcohol poisoning were coded as deaths from alcoholism at the Swedish National Central Bureau of Statistics.

A proportion of the cases included in the Swedish records under the heading deaths from alcoholism were thus originally considered to be alcohol poisoning deaths; the change in classification occurred in connection with coding. Hence, the diagnostic difference between Finland and Sweden is due not only to a difference in diagnostic practice, but depends also on a difference in coding practice.

Comment

The group of deaths from alcohol poisoning and that of deaths from alcoholism differed in Finland and were similar in Sweden with regard to alcohol-related factors. Alcoholism was preferred as a diagnosis particularly at the National Institute of Forensic Medicine in Stockholm and in codifying the underlying cause of death.

It should be borne in mind that the establishment of the cause of death implies integration of all the available data on the case. The variables tested do not represent all significant information used in identifying causes of deaths. On the other hand, these variables characterize the alcohol consumption and its effects in a more condensed form than any other variables that might be selected. They are beyond doubt of essential importance in the determination of the causes of alcohol-related deaths.

The information obtained concerning the places where the death certificates had been written together with the statistical classification of the cases strongly suggests that two parallel diagnostic traditions exist in Sweden. Alcoholism is used in Stockholm and alcohol poisoning in other places as a label for largely similar cases. This view is supported by Swedish investigations on alcohol-related mortality. In a report from the National Institute of Forensic Medicine in Lund the term intoxication with ethyl alcohol is used for cases in which large amounts of alcohol are demonstrated post mortem (Saldeen and Johansson 1967). On the other hand, in studies of delirium tremens patients and vagrant males in Stockholm it has been stated that alcoholism usually is, and according to the rules drawn up by WHO should be, considered the underlying cause of death in the presence of pertinent evidence, although this is likely to result in the underestimation of certain other causes of death, such as liver cirrhosis, pancreatitis and accidents (Salum 1972, 90–91, Alström et al. 1975). In a study on mortality among vagrant males in Stockholm, the underlying cause of death was re-evaluated in 38 psychiatric cases. Alcohol psychosis had been indicated as the underlying cause of death in one of these, drug abuse in two and alcoholism in 35. On re-evaluation it was concluded that death was caused by acute alcohol poisoning in 10 of the latter (Alström et al. 1975). These reports corroborate the present conclusions as to the existence of discrepancies in diagnostic practice.

Indirect evidence of diagnostic differences

It may also be suspected that causes of death other than alcoholism are sometimes confused with alcohol poisoning. The most likely alternatives are other alcohol-related causes. Moreover, sudden death from an unknown cause may be associated with alcohol consumption. The relationship between mortality from these causes and alcohol poisoning mortality will be analysed in this section.

Methods

It was assumed that the mortality from alcohol poisoning is higher in Finland than in the other Nordic countries because alcohol poisoning deaths are classified under other causes of death more often in the other Nordic countries than in Finland. The validity of this assumption was tested by indirect inference. If (1) the frequency of a given pathological finding is lower in some other Nordic group of alcohol poisoning deaths than in Finland and if (2) in the country in question the recorded mortality from this abnormality is higher than in Finland, it may be considered likely that the assumption is valid. The validity of the assumption cannot be considered proved even if the above-mentioned criteria are fulfilled, since the inference is indirect. However, the comparison implies a simple and practicable way of clarifying the possible presence of diagnostic differences and their nature.

The comparison will be limited to mortality among males, as this constitutes most of the total mortality from alcohol poisoning. Moreover, only the population aged 15 and over will be considered, since this is the group mainly exposed to the risks connected with alcohol.

Results

The mortality from certain causes of death in each of the four Nordic countries during the period 1967—1971 was calculated per one million person-years (Table 15). These mortality rates were compared with the frequency of the corresponding pathological findings in autopsied cases in the alcohol poisoning groups in the different Nordic countries.

Alcohol poisoning may be confused with *alcohol psychosis*. However, the mortality rates for alcohol psychosis were so small in the Nordic countries (Table 15) that they cannot include any significant number of deaths which in fact were due to alcohol poisoning.

Bronchitis was observed in 46 per cent of male alcohol poisoning deaths in Finland, in 28 per cent in Denmark, in 9 per cent in Sweden and in 4 per cent in Norway. In contrast, the mortality from acute and undefined bronchitis was higher in Swedish and Danish males than in Finnish males (Table 15). This may imply that some of the deaths attributed in Sweden and Denmark to bronchitis might have been classified as alcohol poisoning in Finland. On the other hand, the deaths from bronchitis were not so numerous that a possible diagnostic confusion would explain the inter-country differences in alcohol poisoning mortality to any important extent.

The mortality from *liver cirrhosis* was clearly higher in Sweden and Denmark than in Finland and Norway. The frequency of liver cirrhosis among the alcohol poisoning deaths ranged from 0 to 2 per cent in the different countries. As there was practically no inter-country difference in frequency for this pathological finding, diagnostic confusion does not seem likely with regard to cirrhosis.

The importance of *fatty liver* must also be considered, since the ICD includes fatty infiltration and cirrhosis of the liver in the same cause-of-death category (WHO 1967, 219). In Sweden, deaths have been attributed to liver cirrhosis on the evidence of fatty infiltration (Alström et al. 1975). However, the proportion of fatty liver cases among males who had died of alcohol poisoning was smaller in Finland (42 per cent) than in the other Nordic countries (45—56 per cent). It is therefore not probable that alcohol poisoning deaths in the latter countries had been classified as deaths from cirrhosis to any notable extent.

The frequency of *pancreatitis* was higher in the Finnish group of alcohol poisoning deaths (5 per cent) than in the other Nordic countries (1—2 per cent). This difference cannot be attributed to more frequent classification of pancreatitis as the underlying cause of death in these countries unless it can be shown that their mortality rates for pancreatitis are higher. The Finnish and Swedish figures are of the same magnitude, however, and higher than the Danish and Norwegian figures (Table 15).

Table 15. Male mortality in some cause-of-death categories in the Nordic countries 1967–1971

Underlying cause of death (code number, ICD, Eighth Revision)	Mortality (per one million person-years) Number of deaths in parentheses			
	Denmark	Finland	Norway	Sweden
Alcohol psychosis (291)	2 (15)	1 (12)	3 (22)	4 (60)
Alcoholism (303)	5 (48)	31 (259)	13 (93)	48 (758)
Acute bronchitis and bronchiolitis (466)	72 (132)	22 (36)	7 (10)	67 (209)
Bronchitis NUD (490)	53 (97)	15 (25)	26 (37)	29 (90)
Liver cirrhosis (571)	113 (1037)	69 (576)	65 (468)	119 (1868)
Acute pancreatitis* (577)	13 (116)	33 (273)	11 (49)	37 (582)
Senility without mention of psychosis (794)	25 (226)	24 (203)	133 (957)	41 (649)
Sudden death (cause unknown) (795)	71 (655)	17 (141)	484 (3477)	9 (134)
Alcohol poisoning (E 860)	8 (69)	123 (1034)	29 (211)	19 (293)
Excessive cold (E 901)	3 (26)	13 (107)	6 (45)	3 (54)
Accidental drowning (E 910)	33 (304)	97 (815)	65 (465)	44 (686)
Inhalation and ingestion of food causing obstruction or suffocation (E 911)	6 (58)	11 (93)	3 (24)	9 (137)
Suicide and self-inflicted injury by solid or liquid substances (E 950)	88 (810)	49 (411)	24 (170)	94 (1480)

* Norwegian data from 1969–1971

Cases which are in reality due to alcohol poisoning may be concealed in certain ill-defined cause-of-death categories. In the group *sudden death due to unknown cause* Norway had markely higher mortality rates than the other Nordic countries. The same applies to *senile marasmus*. The absolute numbers of deaths were also large in these groups. Some authors have pointed out that alcoholics may die suddenly for no ostensible reason (Salum 1972, 99; Kuller et al. 1966).

Sudden death from an unknown cause appears to be a diagnosis which might conceal deaths from alcohol poisoning in Norway. The Norwegian mortality rates by age groups in this cause-of-death category increased steadily in 1970, and this age-related increase was by and large exponential. No particular peak, which might include deaths from alcohol poisoning, was observed. On the other hand, the absence of a peak does not necessarily imply that the group of sudden deaths from an unknown cause cannot include a notable number of alcohol poisoning deaths, as the majority of these deaths occur at ages between 30 and 69 years, ages which were very numerously represented in the group of sudden deaths (380 cases in 1970).

The effects of alcohol are aggravated by *cold,* which may be a factor of importance in the choice between diagnostic alternatives. However, among the males who had died of alcohol poisoning the deleterious effects of frostbite were detected in only 5 per cent in Norway, 3 per cent in Denmark, 2 per cent in Finland and 1 per cent in Sweden. No obvious differences in the frequency of signs of frostbite were observed. Moreover, mortality from the corresponding cause, excessive cold, was higher in Finland than in the other Nordic countries (Table 15).

Drowning is often associated with alcohol use. Among the males who had died of alcohol poisoning, drowning was indicated as a contributory cause only in Sweden (2 per cent). As the mortality from drowning was higher in Finland than in any other Nordic country (Table 15), it may be stated that this cause of death is of minor importance from the standpoint of diagnostic differences in the assumed direction.

Suffocating vomit in the lower respiratory tract was a more frequent finding in the Swedish group of alcohol poisoning deaths (16 per cent) than in the other national groups (8—9 per cent). The corresponding cause-of-death category, *inhalation of food causing suffocation,* was scantily represented in all of the Nordic countries and is therefore of no interest in analysing diagnostic differences.

The category of *suicide by poisoning with solid or liquid substances* is highly represented (Table 15) and might include alcohol poisonings, if views on the intentional use of alcohol for destructive purposes differed substantially from one Nordic country to another. However, sucide by alcohol alone is a rare phenomenon (Harenko 1968). It is more likely that poisoning caused by alcohol

Table 16. Drugs observed post-mortem among autopsied males who died of alcohol poisoning

Drug group	Denmark Per cent	Finland Per cent	Norway Per cent	Sweden [a] Per cent
Barbiturates	12	3	3	17
Other soporifics	2	0	–	2
Psychopharmaceutics	2	4	1	11
Analgesics	2	3	–	7
Total	18	10	4	37
Number of autopsies	43	296	112	211

and drugs in combination is diagnosed as suicide. If this were a noteworthy diagnostic alternative to alcohol poisoning, drugs ought to be found at post-mortem examination in a larger proportion of Finnish alcohol poisoning deaths than in the other Nordic countries. However, the proportion of cases where drugs were discovered at autopsy was smaller only in Norway than in Finland; in both Sweden and Denmark, drugs were detected at autopsy in a much larger proportion of cases than in Finland (Table 16).

Comment

Some cases have been described in which alcohol poisoning was erroneously diagnosed in Sweden. A diagnosis of liver cirrhosis has sometimes been made on the basis of acute alcohol poisoning and one elevated serum transaminase value (Wadman et al. 1971). One death statistically recorded under the heading delirium was considered to be due in fact to acute alcohol poisoning (Salum 1972, 98). On comparing the frequency of pathological findings in males who had died of alcohol poisoning with the mortality from the corresponding causes of death, no consistent observations suggesting any diagnostic confusion were made. Therefore, the preponderance of alcohol poisoning deaths in Finland compared with the other Nordic countries cannot be explained by differences in diagnostic practice. The comparison shows that the instances of a deviating classification as described in the literature are exceptions rather than the rule.

VIII
IMPLICATIONS OF DRINKING HABITS

For the purposes of the present study, it was assumed that drinking is more violent in Finland than in the other Nordic countries and that this is reflected in the higher degree of intoxication produced. Phenomena which could be expected to prove the validity of this assumption were analysed.

Motives for drinking

The records were scrutinized for information on the motives behind drinking which terminated in fatal alcohol poisoning. Motive is here used in the wide sense of the word, meaning any reason or inducement. It was assumed that drinking would be induced for instance by drinking competitions, betting on one's drinking prowess and a desire to celebrate release from various enclosed institutions. However, a clear motive for drinking could only be found in five cases in the Finnish and one in the Norwegian material.

Mortality on holidays

It was assumed that uncontrolled, though infrequent, drinking resulting in fatal alcohol poisoning would be reflected in increased mortality rates for public holidays. This assumption was tested with regard to New Year, May Day and Midsummer Day. The statistical significance was tested by means of binomial distribution (Hollander and Wolfe 1973, 16), assuming as the null hypothesis that the probability of death is the same on each day of the year. The number of holiday deaths was low (Table 17). However, the death rates for alcohol poisoning were higher than expected on Midsummer Day in Finland ($p < .01$) and on May Day ($p < .01$) and Midsummer Day ($p < 0.5$) in Sweden. The fact that violent drinking was not notably reflected in the mortality rates for public holidays suggests that in the groups investigated uncontrolled drinking was not infrequent on other days.

Table 17. Deaths from alcohol poisoning or alcoholism which occurred on holidays

Holiday	Alcohol poisoning				Alcoholism	
	Denmark	Finland	Norway	Sweden[s]	Finland	Sweden[s]
New Year (Dec. 31-Jan.2)	–	2	–	1	–	1
May Day (April 30-May 2)	2	3	2	7**	2	1
Midsummer Day (June 20–24)	1	9**	5	7*	1	–

* $.01 \leqq p < .05$ ** $p < .01$ Binomial test (Hollander and Wolfe 1973, 16)

Postmortal blood ethanol concentration

The blood ethanol concentration determined post mortem reflects the premortal concentration. Postmortal chemical changes do not essentially affect the validity of the values obtained as a measure of ingested ethanol (Appendix 2). The postmortal ethanol concentration was therefore studied as an indicator of the violence of drinking.

The mean postmortal blood ethanol concentration was highest in the Finnish group of alcohol poisoning deaths, 3.2 per mille. The corresponding value for the Norwegian group was 3.0 per mille, while a mean value of 2.6 per mille was noted in the Danish and Swedish groups. The distributions of the values were unimodal and symmetric (Table 18); a small supernumerary peak (for concentrations of 1.00–1.49 per mille) was observed only in the Swedish group. The averages of the postmortal blood ethanol concentrations were, therefore, adequately expressed by the mean values.

Due to the similarity in shape of the distributions and the similarity in standard deviations (Table 18), the statistical significance of the differences between the groups was tested by the two-sided *t*-test. This revealed a high significance ($p = .000–.013$), except for the difference between the Swedish and Danish alcohol poisoning groups and the difference between the alcohol poisoning and alcoholism groups in Sweden (Table 19).

Ethanol concentrations in excess of 5 per mille were very rare; a concentration between 2 and 5 per mille was noted in most cases. Cases with an ethanol concentration of 3 per mille or more constituted 79 per cent in Finland, 58 per cent in Norway, 39 per cent in Sweden and 38 per cent in Denmark of all alcohol poisoning deaths in which the concentration was determined by the enzymatic or gas chromatographic method. Among those who had died of

Table 18. Post-mortem blood ethanol concentration measured by an enzymatic or gas chromatographic method in persons who died of alcohol poisoning or alcoholism

	Alcohol poisoning				Alcoholism	
Blood ethanol concentration (per mille)	Denmark Per cent	Finland Per cent	Norway Per cent	Sweden Per cent	Finland Per cent	Sweden Per cent
0.01–0.49	3	2	4	0	6	4
0.50–0.99	6	2	—	2	14	13
1.00–1.49	8	1	4	13	17	9
1.50–1.99	14	4	3	11	20	13
2.00–2.49	14	9	10	16	23	17
2.50–2.99	17	12	21	19	11	15
3.00–3.49	22	30	28	19	6	17
3.50–3.99	9	24	22	13	2	4
4.00–4.49	6	12	7	4	—	4
4.50–4.99	—	3	1	2	—	2
5.00–5.49	2	1	—	1	—	2
5.50–5.99	—	0	—	—	—	—
6.00–6.49	—	0	—	—	—	—
Total	101	100	100	100	99	100
Number of cases	65	305	123	213	64	47
Arithmetic mean	2.56	3.21	2.96	2.60	1.78	2.32
Standard deviation	1.06	0.94	0.94	0.96	0.86	1.19

Table 19. Statistical significance of the differences in post-mortem ethanol concentration (per mille) determined by an enzymatic or gas chromatographic method (p-value)

	Denmark, alcohol poisoning	Finland, alcohol poisoning	Norway, alcohol poisoning	Sweden, alcohol poisoning	Finland, alcoholism
Finland, alcohol poisoning	.000				
Norway, alcohol poisoning	.009	.013			
Sweden, alcohol poisoning	.774	.000	.001		
Finland, alcoholism	.000	.000	.000	.000	
Sweden, alcoholism	.263	.000	.000	.084	.006

Two-sided t-test

alcoholism a concentration of over 3 per mille was noted in 8 per cent of cases in Finland and in 30 per cent of cases in Sweden.

As the Swedish material included a relatively larger number of cases in which drugs were detected in addition to alcohol, the postmortal ethanol concentrations were also analysed after exclusion of those cases in which drugs had been found. The mean values thus calculated were 3.3 per mille in Finland, 3.0 in Norway, 2.9 in Sweden and 2.7 per mille in Denmark. The inter-country differences and the magnitude of the mean values remained more or less unaffected.

Alcohol consumption at the Skid Row level

When the drinking habits of those who had died of alcohol poisoning in the different Nordic countries were compared, Skid Row alcoholism was established as being most common in Finland (Table 20). The highest statistical significance was noted for the difference between the Finns and the Swedes, the next highest for the difference between the Finns and the Danes, while the difference between the Finns and the Norwegians was slight (Table 21). It is noteworthy that the proportion of Skid Row alcoholics was highly significantly larger in the Finnish group of deaths from alcoholism than in any other group.

Alcoholism on the Skid Row level was closely connected with the consumption of industrial alcohol products. According to the data collected by the police, industrial alcohol had been used during the fatal drinking session in 29 per cent of cases in Finland, in 12 per cent in Denmark, in 9 per cent in Sweden

Table 20. Drinking habits among persons who died of alcohol poisoning or alcoholism

	Alcohol poisoning				Alcoholism	
Drinking habits	Denmark Per cent	Finland Per cent	Norway Per cent	Sweden [s] Per cent	Finland Per cent	Sweden [s] Per cent
Total abstainer	–	–	2	1	–	–
Moderate user	3	2	2	11	–	5
Heavy user	74	60	71	76	41	82
Skid Row alcoholic	22	38	25	13	59	13
Total	99	100	100	101	100	100
Number of cases	89	168	55	160	103	77
No information	17	160	183	144	15	24

Table 21. Statistical significance of the differences in frequency of Skid Row alcoholism (p-value)

	Denmark, alcohol poisoning	Finland, alcohol poisoning	Norway, alcohol poisoning	Sweden, alcohol poisoning	Finland, alcoholism
Finland, alcohol poisoning	.011				
Norway, alcohol poisoning	.681	.088			
Sweden, alcohol poisoning	.057	.000	.033		
Finland, alcoholism	.000	.001	.000	.000	
Sweden, alcoholism	.113	.000	.067	.975	.000

Chi-square contingency test, 1 df

and in 5 per cent in Norway (Table 22). The chemical examinations performed at autopsy revealed industrial alcohol in a larger number of cases in Finland (16 per cent) than in Sweden (11 per cent), Denmark (8 per cent) or Norway (5 per cent) (Table 23). As was to be expected, the use of alcohol substitutes was more common among the Skid Row alcoholics than in the remainder of the material. The data on previous drinking habits and the data on the use of industrial alcohol products all show that a chronic alcohol consumption resulting in a decline in social status was more common among those who had died of alcohol poisoning in Finland than in the other Nordic countries.

According to police reports, 63 (53 per cent) out of 119 subjects in the Nordic countries regarded as Skid Row alcoholics had drunk industrial alcohol. The corresponding figure for the remaining 353 deceased persons whose previous drinking habits were known was 51 (14 per cent). Hence, industrial alcohol products were more frequently resorted to by Skid Row alcoholics than by other drinkers. The same finding was arrived at by means of chemical examinations performed at autopsy. Industrial alcohol was found in 30 of the 119 Skid Row alcoholics and in 31 of the remaining 353 cases.

A correlation was observed between the frequency of Skid Row alcoholism and the frequency of dying out of doors. Death had occurred outdoors in 31 per cent of Skid Row cases in Finland, in 24 per cent in Norway, in 16 per cent in Denmark and in 13 per cent in Sweden. In Finland, about two-thirds of the Skid

Table 22. Industrial alcohols reported to have been ingested by persons who died of alcohol poisoning or alcoholism

	Alcohol poisoning				Alcoholism	
Type of industrial alcohol	Denmark Per cent	Finland Per cent	Norway Per cent	Sweden S Per cent	Finland Per cent	Sweden S Per cent
Technical ethanol products	8	26	3	0	20	–
Methanol	–	1	–	–	–	–
Isopropanol	–	2	–	–	–	–
Methanol and ethanol in combination	4	0	2	9	–	8
Ethanol and isopropanol in combination	–	0	–	–	–	–
Total	12	29	5	9	20	8
Number of cases	106	328	238	304	118	101

Table 23. Industrial alcohols chemically demonstrated among autopsied cases of alcohol poisoning or alcoholism

	Alcohol poisoning				Alcoholism	
Type of industrial alcohol	Denmark Per cent	Finland Per cent	Norway Per cent	Sweden S Per cent	Finland Per cent	Sweden S Per cent
Technical ethanol products	–	12	–	–	9	–
Methanol	8	2	5	11	–	8
Isopropanol	–	2	–	–	2	–
Total	8	16	5	11	11	8
Number of autopsies	61	317	125	238	86	77

Row alcoholics had died outdoors, as opposed to about only one-fifth of the other victims of fatal alcohol poisoning. The corresponding ratios for those whose death was attributed to alcoholism were about three-fifths and one-tenth.

Mortality of Finnish immigrants in Sweden

The material provided an opportunity for comparing the alcohol-related mortality of Finns and Swedes under circumstances which may be assumed to be similar as regards diagnostics and thoroughness of cause-of-death inquiries, i.e. by comparing the mortality rates for Swedes born in Sweden and for Finnish immigrants in Sweden. The average population of Finnish immigrants in Sweden in 1967–1971 was calculated on annual estimates of the average population (Edgren and Wiman 1973, 23). The death rates for alcoholism were calculated on the assumption that the proportions of Swedes and Finnish immigrants among all who had died of alcoholism in Sweden in 1967–1971 were the same as in the sample of deaths for 1969–1971. The significance of the mortality rates was estimated by calculating the 99 per cent confidence limits of the Poisson distribution.

The alcohol poisoning mortality of the Finnish immigrants was almost twice that of the Swedes (Table 24). However, as the number of Finnish immigrants among the deceased was only 15, the 99 per cent confidence intervals were wide and overlapped.

As regards mortality from alcoholism, there was a clear difference between the Swedes and the Finnish immigrants: 112 per one million person-years among the latter against 17 per one million person-years among the former. The difference was significant ($p < .01$). According to this estimate, the mortality from alcoholism of Finnish immigrants in Sweden was about five times higher than the mortality of the Swedes.

Table 24. Mortality from alcohol poisoning and alcoholism in Swedes and Finnish immigrants in Sweden

	Mortality (per one million person-years) (99 per cent confidence limits)	
	Alcohol poisoning [1]	Alcoholism [2]
Swedes	9 (7–10)	22 (16–28)
Finnish immigrants in Sweden	17 (8–32)	112 (48–220)

[1] All deaths in 1967–1971.
[2] Estimates based on a 20 per cent sample of deaths in 1969–1971.

Comment

The mean postmortal ethanol concentration was higher in the Finnish group of alcohol poisoning deaths than in the other Nordic groups. This does not necessarily mean that the premortal maximum blood ethanol concentration was also higher in the Finnish group. On the other hand, there is no reason to assume that the elimination of ethanol from the blood is slower, or that the interval between the maximum blood ethanol concentration and death is shorter, in Finns than in Swedes, Danes or Norwegians. The higher postmortal mean ethanol concentration seems to constitute evidence, although indirectly, of more uncontrolled drinking among those who died of alcohol poisoning in Finland.

The connection between frequent intoxication and a large over-all consumption explains the present observation that mortality from alcohol poisoning on public holidays did not appreciably exceed the mortality on other days. The distribution of the death risk over the days of the year presumably follows the distribution of heavy drinking sessions, and for a heavy drinker the holidays are not numerous enough for such drinking. However, as the present investigation revealed a significantly higher mortality on certain public holidays than expected, it may be assumed that to some extent drinking among heavy consumers follows the general drinking rhythm. This assumption is compatible with a report on the drinking habits of Finnish alcoholics (Ahlström-Laakso 1975, 113).

The proportion of Skid Row alcoholics among all those who had died of alcohol poisoning was clearly larger in Finland than in the other Nordic countries. It seems likely that the label Skid Row alcoholic would also have been appropriate in a number of those cases in which information on previous drinking habits was lacking. In a study carried out by Alha (1970a), 70 new Skid Row cases came to light in a questionnaire distributed to medicolegal experts in 1967. Some cases of Skid Row alcoholism, however, have probably also remained unrecognized in the other Nordic countries. As the identification of Skid Row cases is based on police reports in all these countries, it may be assumed that the same degree of under-estimation is involved in all of them and that it may therefore be considered appropriate to discuss the inter-country differences on the basis of the present results. The conclusion seems justified that Skid Row alcoholics are relatively more numerous in Finland than in the other Nordic countries among persons who die of alcohol poisoning. This conclusion is also supported by the higher frequency of the consumption of industrial alcohol products by the Finnish victims of fatal alcohol poisoning and the larger proportion of subjects who had died out of doors.

The larger proportion of Skid Row alcoholics among the victims of fatal alcohol poisoning in Finland compared with Sweden seems to be due mainly to the fact that Skid Row alcoholism is more common in Finland. It is difficult to estimate the number of Skid Row alcoholics owing both to the vagrant nature of their lives and to the lack of a precise definition of this kind of alcoholism. However, roughly calculated on the total populations during the study period there seemed to be about four times more Skid Row alcoholics in Finland than in Sweden. On the basis of questionnaires answered by the police it was estimated that about 8 000 Finnish subjects used alcohol substitutes in 1967 and in 1969, and that somewhat over half of these drank industrial alcohol products habitually and the remainder occasionally (Pöysä and Mäkelä 1970). In Sweden, the number of alcoholics who drink industrial T-spirits has been estimated at about 4 000 (Jacobson and Eriksson 1972). The number of alcoholics of no fixed abode in Norway has been estimated at some 5 000 (Brun-Gulbrandsen, personal communication 1977).

The industrial alcohol product most frequently used in Finland — T-spirits* — contains no methanol, whereas the corresponding Swedish product contains about 2—5 volume per cent methanol (Jackobson and Eriksson 1972). This difference in composition explains why positive salicylaldehyde and vanillin reactions were generally observed in those who had died of alcohol poisoning in Finland, while both methanol and ethanol were often found in the tissues of the deceased in Sweden.

Mortality from alcoholism among the Finnish immigrants in Sweden was about 400 per cent higher than the corresponding figure for the Swedes. Bearing in mind that the subjects who died of alcoholism in Sweden were fundamentally similar to those who died of alcohol poisoning, and that alcoholism was commonly indicated as the cause of death in the Stockholm area (pp. 74—79), where the majority of the deaths among Finnish immigrants occurred, it seems reasonable to assume that the alcohol poisoning mortality rate of the Finnish immigrants in Sweden was of the same magnitude as that of the Finns living in Finland.

The present results do not permit any definite statement with regard to the cause of the higher alcohol poisoning mortality among the Finnish immigrants in Sweden compared with the Swedes. However, the assumption that drinking habits are the main determinant of the differences in mortality is supported by the fact that immigrants as a rule stick to inveterate cultural habits. This assumption is further corroborated by observations indicating that alcoholics immigrated from Finland have harder drinking habits and a higher frequency of delirium tremens and acute hallucinosis than native-born Swedish alcoholics (Lindfors 1976).

* Available for sale from 1967 to 1972 (Korvikealkoholitoimikunnan... 1973, 8—10 and 21).

IX
PATHOLOGICAL FINDINGS IN DEATHS FROM ALCOHOL POISONING AND ALCOHOLISM

The same factors that are responsible for the variation in mortality from alcohol poisoning may also affect the frequency of pathological organic changes. The frequency of such changes may be connected with (1) the level of previous alcohol consumption. Alcohol may have (a) a direct toxic effect or (b) it may cause organic changes indirectly, i.e. by its harmful effects on the metabolism and nutritional state of the organism. Drinking may be associated (2) with factors which are not directly due to alcohol, but correlate with it and affect mortality. The drinker's way of life and dietary habits, e.g. smoking, constitute such factors. Organic changes may also (3) result from causes other than alcohol consumption or alcohol-related factors.

Pulmonary findings

Results

Bronchitis was clearly more frequently associated with death from alcohol poisoning and alcoholism in Finland than in the other Nordic countries (Table 25). The differences between the Finnish and the other alcohol poisoning groups, and the differences between the Danish group of alcohol poisoning and the corresponding Swedish and Norwegian groups, were significant (Table 26). Pneumonia was an occasional finding in all alcohol poisoning groups, but not so rare in the alcoholic groups. Active tuberculosis was rare in all groups.

The aspiration of gastric contents may cause inflammation of the bronchi. However, aspiration occurred in the total material in only about 7 per cent of those cases in which bronchitis was observed at autopsy. Thus, bronchitis was due to some cause other than aspiration in the majority of cases.

Table 25. Pathological pulmonary findings among autopsied cases of alcohol poisoning or alcoholism

	Alcohol poisoning				Alcoholism	
Finding	Denmark Per cent	Finland Per cent	Norway Per cent	Sweden[s] Per cent	Finland Per cent	Sweden[s] Per cent
Bronchitis	21	46	6	9	45	13
Pneumonia	2	3	1	3	13	9
Active tuberculosis	2	1	—	—	2	—
Number of autopsies	61	317	125	238	86	77

Table 26. Statistical significance of the differences in frequency of bronchitis (p-value)

	Denmark, alcohol poisoning	Finland, alcohol poisoning	Norway, alcohol poisoning	Sweden, alcohol poisoning	Finland, alcoholism
Finland, alcohol poisoning	.000				
Norway, alcohol poisoning	.003	.000			
Sweden, alcohol poisoning	.006	.000	.418		
Finland, alcoholism	.003	.906	.000	.000	
Sweden, alcoholism	.193	.000	.111	.286	.000

Chi-square contingency test, 1 df

Comment

Alcohol predisposes the drinker to pulmonary disease, and morbidity seems to be directly related to the degree of exposure to the harmful influence. In experiments on mice it was shown that the capacity of the lungs to eliminate pneumococci decreased when the animals were given alcohol (Stillman 1924), and the larger the dose of ethanol per kg of body weight, the more it decreased (Auerbach-Rubin and Ottolenghi-Nightingale 1971). The same observation has been reported with regard to staphylococci (Louria 1963, Green and Kass 1964). The mechanisms responsible for the deterioration of the bacteria-eliminating capacity are known. Alcohol depresses the reflex that closes the glottis, and this promotes the aspiration of the mucin necessary for the development of pneumonia (Nungester and Klepser 1938). The motility of the cilia which remove foreign bodies from the lungs slows up with rising blood ethanol concentration (Laurenzi and Guarneri 1966). Alcohol impairs chemotaxis in both rats (Klepser and Nungester 1939) and humans during intoxication, but not during abstinence (Brayton et al. 1970). It has been shown that alcohol inhibits myelopoiesis in vitro (Tisman and Herbert 1973), and leukopenic conditions have been observed in alcoholics (Liu 1973). In contrast, alcohol does not affect the capacity of human polymorphonuclear leukocytes to phagocytose bacteria or to kill phagocytosed bacteria intracellularly (Brayton et al. 1970).

Furthermore, chronic, heavy alcohol consumption is accompanied by undernourishment. This impairs the competence of the thymus- and bone marrow-dependent immune systems (Law et al. 1973).

The correlation between alcohol consumption and pulmonary disease appears in the mortality rates. It has been shown that mortality from pneumonia is higher in clinically defined alcoholics than in the general population (Sundby 1967, Schmidt and de Lint 1972). A higher total mortality rate from pneumonia and influenza has also been observed in alcoholics compared with the general population (Brenner 1967). In the light of these results on the lack of resistance to infection and the mortality from lung diseases among alcoholics, it seems likely that the excessive mortality rate is due in part at least to the effects of alcohol.

A high frequency of pulmonary disease may also be due to factors other than alcohol. Smoking, in particular, may be responsible. Chronic obstructive pulmonary disease has been commonly found in alcoholics who smoke and rarely in non-smokers (Rankin et al. 1969). Heavy drinkers also smoke a great many cigarettes (Friberg et al. 1973, Myrhed 1974, 34–39, Friedman et al. 1974, Maletzky and Klotter 1974). Alcoholics smoke more than other psychiatric patients, irrespective of personality variations in the extroversion-introversion dimension (Ayers et al. 1976).

Since smoking and drinking correlate in the general population, it may be assumed that heavy drinkers are, almost without exception, heavy smokers. If this is so, variation due to smoking is not likely to occur to any appreciable extent among heavy drinkers. Evidence in this direction was put forward in an investigation on the pulmonary function of 23 patients treated for "acute alcoholism" at a detoxification department; a group who drank a good deal and another group who drank a great deal smoked about the same number of cigarettes (Emirgil et al. 1974). Chronic bronchitis was observed in 21 of these patients, and spirometry revealed chronic obstructive lung disease in two-thirds. The results suggest that alcohol exercises an effect that is independent of smoking. Banner (1973) found that the diffusion capacity of carbon monoxide was further reduced in alcoholics than was anticipated on the basis of their smoking habits and that this decrease correlated with the duration of uncontrolled drinking. This report also seems to indicate that alcohol may have a toxic effect on the lungs which is independent of smoking.

Bearing in mind the results of investigations on the etiology of pulmonary diseases and on the mechanisms of the harmful effects of alcohol on the capacity of the lungs to eliminate bacteria, it seems probable that the high frequency of bronchitis and pneumonia in the Finnish deaths from alcohol poisoning and alcoholism can be ascribed to the consumption of large quantities of alcohol. The role of smoking as a factor enhancing the probability of pulmonary disease in heavy drinkers cannot be assessed on the basis of the present material. Smoking may have some significance, but the effects of alcohol alone perhaps suffice to explain the differences observed.

Suffocation by aspirated gastric contents

Results

Gastric contents in amounts sufficient to block the airways were found in the lungs in a larger number of cases in the Swedish groups of deaths from alcohol poisoning and alcoholism than in any other national group (Table 27). The most significant differences were observed between the Swedish and Finnish alcohol poisonings, the Swedish and Norwegian alcohol poisonings, the Swedish deaths from alcoholism and the Finnish deaths from alcohol poisoning, and between the Swedish deaths from alcoholism and the Norwegian deaths from alcohol poisoning (Table 28). On the other hand, the differences between the groups were slight with regard to the presence of small, non-obstructing quantities of aspirated gastric contents.

It was assumed that the frequent occurrence of suffocation by aspirated gastric contents among those who had died of alcohol poisoning in Sweden was due to the high proportion of poisoning caused by drugs and alcohol in combination. Therefore, the deaths caused by drug and alcohol poisoning and the deaths from alcohol poisoning alone in Sweden were compared with regard to the presence of vomit blocking the airways. This finding was made in 22 per cent of 78 combined drug and alcohol poisonings and in only 11 per cent of 226 pure alcohol poisonings. Hence, aspiration of gastric contents was more common among those who had ingested both alcohol and drugs. However, drug use was

Table 27. Occurrence of gastric contents in lower respiratory tract among autopsied cases of alcohol poisoning or alcoholism

Amount of gastric contents	Alcohol poisoning				Alcoholism	
	Denmark Per cent	Finland Per cent	Norway Per cent	Sweden[s] Per cent	Finland Per cent	Sweden[s] Per cent
Slight	7	4	8	5	2	4
Obstructing	8	9	7	17	8	19
Number of autopsies	61	317	125	238	86	77

Table 28. Statistical significance of the differences in frequency of aspirated gastric contents causing respiratory obstruction (p-value)

	Denmark, alcohol poisoning	Finland, alcohol poisoning	Norway, alcohol poisoning	Sweden, alcohol poisoning	Finland, alcoholism
Finland, alcohol poisoning	.813				
Norway, alcohol poisoning	x	.511			
Sweden, alcohol poisoning	.093	.007	.011		
Finland, alcoholism	x	.772	.799	.050	
Sweden, alcoholism	.061	.010	.009	.592	.034

Chi-square contingency test, 1 df

involved in somewhat less than half of the cases in which the aspiration of gastric contents had caused suffocation. Only in the Swedish material was a clear connection between drug use and suffocation by aspirated gastric contents observed.

Comment

Suffocation by aspirated gastric contents was the immediate cause of death in almost one-fifth of the Swedish material, as opposed to one-tenth in the other

Nordic countries. A correlation between suffocation by aspirated gastric contents and poisoning caused by the combined use of drugs and alcohol was observed in Sweden, but not in the other countries. Factors favouring aspiration may be more common in Sweden, but there is no straightforward explanation for the phenomenon in question.

Myocardial findings

Results

Myocardial abnormalities were recorded by using the classification introduced by Alha and Tenhu (Alha 1970a). Myofibrosis was the most common finding. It was clearly most frequent in the Swedish group of alcohol poisonings (Table 29). The frequency of myofibrosis was significantly higher in this group than in the Finnish and Norwegian groups of deaths from alcohol poisoning and in the Finnish and Swedish groups of deaths attributed to alcoholism (Table 30). On the other hand, myofibrosis was a less frequent finding in the Danish group of alcohol poisonings than in the Finnish and Norwegian groups. Hypertrophy and myocardial dilatation were more frequent in the Finnish and Swedish alcohol poisoning groups than in the other groups (Table 29).

Hypertrophy and dilatation were present in so few cases in most groups that the statistical significance of the differences between these groups was not tested. The most significant difference was noted between the Finnish and the Norwegian alcohol poisoning groups ($p = .033$). Myocardosis, fatty degeneration and fatty infiltration were only found in the Finnish material (Table 29). Infarction scars, endocarditis, cardiomyopathy, pericarditis and cor pulmonale were very infrequent in all groups.

Comment

Myofibrosis was clearly a more common finding in those who had died of alcohol poisoning in Sweden than in any other group. Myocardosis was a common finding in the Finnish group of alcohol poisonings, and even more common in the alcoholism group. In general, the differences in other myocardial abnormalities were of minor importance.

Alha (1970a) analysed the myocardial findings in 193 Finnish subjects who had died of alcohol poisoning in 1967. When the present Finnish material of alcohol poisoning deaths is compared with Alha's series, the distribution of myocardial abnormalities is found to be similar (Table 31). The frequency of pathological myocardial findings, therefore, seems very constant.

Table 29. Pathological myocardial findings among autopsied cases of alcohol poisoning or alcoholism

Finding	Alcohol poisoning				Alcoholism	
	Denmark Per cent	Finland Per cent	Norway Per cent	Sweden [s] Per cent	Finland Per cent	Sweden [s] Per cent
Old infarction scar	2	3	—	1	—	—
Myofibrosis	3	22	19	36	22	21
Hypertrophy and dilatation	3	8	2	7	3	3
Endocarditis	—	3	—	—	1	—
Cardiomyopathy	—	—	—	1	1	1
Pericarditis	—	1	—	1	—	—
Cor pulmonale	3	1	2	—	2	—
Myocardosis	—	8	—	—	26	—
Total	11	46	23	46	55	25
Number of autopsies	61	317	125	238	86	77

Table 30. Statistical significance of the differences in frequency of myofibrosis (p-value)

	Denmark, alcohol poisoning	Finland, alcohol poisoning	Norway, alcohol poisoning	Sweden, alcohol poisoning	Finland, alcoholism
Finland, alcohol poisoning	.001				
Norway, alcohol poisoning	.003	.505			
Sweden, alcohol poisoning	.000	.000	.001		
Finland, alcoholism	.001	.998	.608	.017	
Sweden, alcoholism	.002	.803	.784	.012	.838

Chi-square contingency test, 1 df

Table 31. Frequency of myocardial findings in two Finnish series of deaths from alcohol poisoning

	Author (time of investigation)	
Finding	Alha (1967) Per cent	Poikolainen (1968–1971) [1] Per cent
Diffuse myofibrosis or old infarction scar	21	25
Hypertrophy and dilatation [2]	13	9
Endocarditis	3	3
Pericarditis	1	1
Myocardosis	8	6
Number of cases	193	253

[1] Does not include deaths in 1967, which are included in Alha's series.
[2] In Alha's series (1970a) called cardiac insufficiency.
Chi-square contingency test, p = .586, df = 5.

The more frequent occurrence of myocardosis in the alcoholism group, which includes a larger number of Skid Row alcoholics, than in the alcohol poisoning group in Finland seems to indicate that chronic, heavy drinking may be of importance in the pathogenesis of myocardosis. However, it has not been shown that a connection exists between alcohol consumption and non-infectious myocardial disease, corresponding to a patho-anatomical finding that could be defined as myocardosis.

Intra-myocardial accumulation of lipids has been observed in dogs (Regan et al. 1966 and 1974) and mice (Lieber et al. 1966, Burch et al. 1971) given alcohol over a certain period. On the other hand, a larger number of fibrotic changes and a higher degree of inflammation of the myocardium, indicative of infiltration by inflammatory cells, were observed in an autopsy series of chronic alcoholics than in the controls, but fatty infiltration did not occur (Hognestad and Teisberg 1973).

Chronic alcoholism has been found to be frequent in patients with cardiomyopathy (Burch and Giles 1974, 436), but it has been claimed that so far no reliable epidemiological investigation on the relationship between alcohol consumption and cardiac disease has been carried out (Louhija 1972). In Finland, cardiomyopathy is not common in alcoholics; in an unselected series of 100 subjects regarded as chronic alcoholics, not a single case showed signs of cardiomyopathy (Härtel et al. 1969).

Since no correlation has been demonstrated between the use of alcohol and primary cardiac disease characterized by the patho-anatomical finding of myocardosis, fatty degeneration or fatty infiltration, it cannot be concluded that the frequent occurrence of myocardosis in the present Finnish material of alcohol-related deaths was due to alcohol. However, the possible connection between myocardosis and a heavy alcohol intake is certainly worth following up.

In the Swedish material of alcohol poisoning deaths, myofibrosis was found in almost two-fifths of the cases. Although histological investigations were carried out in Sweden somewhat more often than in the other Nordic countries, there seems to be little question of inter-country differences in the diagnosis of myofibrosis, since myofibrosis was markedly less frequent in the group of deaths attributed to alcoholism, which in Sweden was diagnostically similar to the alcohol poisoning group. The difference in question seems a real one, although it is not readily explained.

Ethanol affects the functional capacity of the heart. In experiments on dogs the stroke volume decreased and the left ventricular end-diastolic pressure increased both under the acute influence of alcohol (Regan et al. 1966) and after administration of alcohol over a period of 22 months (Regan et al. 1974). On the other hand, after exposure to the effects of alcohol for 3.5 months, no haemodynamic changes were observed (Pachinger et al. 1973). The development of persistent haemodynamic changes thus seems to require long periods of exposure.

In experimental investigations, changes affecting the function of the heart have been observed in normal subjects (Gould et al. 1973, Ahmed et al. 1973), in cardiac patients with a generally small alcohol consumption (Conway 1968, Gould et al. 1972) and in alcoholics with normal hearts (Regan et al. 1969, Mösslacher 1973). Very small doses of ethanol had no untoward effects on the haemodynamics (Gould et al. 1972, Regan et al. 1969).

The haemodynamic impairment caused by alcohol may enhance the death risk in severe alcohol poisoning. It may be assumed that cardiac disease increases the risk of death from acute alcohol poisoning resulting from uncontrolled drinking, but this assumption cannot be proved. Clarification of this question would require prospective follow-up investigations on both healthy heavy consumers of alcohol and consumers suffering from heart disease who frequently get intoxicated.

Hepatic findings

Results

Fatty infiltration of the liver was observed in about half the number of alcohol poisoning cases (Table 32). The inter-country differences in frequency were slight (Table 32). In contrast, the frequency of this abnormality was markedly higher in the Finnish group of deaths caused by alcoholism than in the Finnish alcohol poisoning group (Table 33).

Table 32. Pathological hepatic findings among autopsied cases of alcohol poisoning or alcoholism

	Alcohol poisoning				Alcoholism	
Finding	Denmark Per cent	Finland Per cent	Norway Per cent	Sweden [s] Per cent	Finland Per cent	Sweden [s] Per cent
Fatty liver	51	43	42	49	85	56
Cirrhosis	—	3	—	3	3	5
Hepatitis	—	—	—	0	—	—
Number of autopsies	61	317	125	238	86	77

Table 33. Statistical significance of the differences in frequency of fatty liver (p-value)

	Denmark, alcohol poisoning	Finland, alcohol poisoning	Norway, alcohol poisoning	Sweden, alcohol poisoning	Finland, alcoholism
Finland, alcohol poisoning	.254				
Norway, alcohol poisoning	.279	.924			
Sweden, alcohol poisoning	.818	.143	.220		
Finland, alcoholism	.000	.000	.000	.000	
Sweden, alcoholism	.436	.041	.063	.308	.000

Chi-square contingency test, 1 df

Liver cirrhosis was found only in a few cases in the various groups. Hepatitis was observed in one Swedish case of alcohol poisoning.

Comment

The frequency of fatty infiltration in the present material of alcohol poisoning deaths was of the same magnitude as that reported in clinical series of alcoholics. In an unselected Finnish series of alcoholics investigated in 1967, the liver was enlarged and/or painful in 52 per cent; an increase in serum transaminases indicating liver damage was observed in about half the cases (Härtel et al. 1969). In a Danish consecutive series of 330 chronic alcoholics admitted for treatment in 1968–1971, liver biopsy revealed fatty infiltration in 64 per cent (Christoffersen and Nielsen 1972).

A notable increase of fat in the liver was observed eight days from the beginning of drinking when the daily dose was 100–170 grams of 100 per cent ethanol and earlier if the daily dose was larger (Feinman and Lieber 1974, 306). The presence of fatty infiltration of the liver may thus be regarded as an indicator of recent heavy alcohol use.

Gastric findings

Results

Acute gastritis was the most common pathological gastric finding. This diagnosis was made if engorgement, erythema and erosions of the gastric mucosa were observed macroscopically. Histological examinations were not usually carried out. Consequently, it was not possible to diagnose chronic, superficial or atrophic gastritis.

When acute gastritis is referred to in the following, it is called gastritis for the sake of brevity. The frequency of this abnormality was highest in the Finnish material (Table 34). The differences between the values for the two Finnish groups and the values for the other national groups were significant, the difference between the Finnish alcohol poisoning group and the Swedish group of deaths from alcoholism excepted (Table 35). The frequency of gastritis was significantly higher in the Swedish alcohol poisoning group than in the Norwegian alcohol poisoning group and in the Swedish group of deaths from alcoholism. The frequency of gastritis was also significantly higher in the Danish alcohol poisoning group than in the corresponding Norwegian group (Table 35). Gastric or duodenal ulcer was found in only a few cases in each group (Table 34). The frequency of gastric resection was slightly higher in the Danish material than in the other groups, all of which showed more or less the same frequency for this finding.

Comment

Gastritis was observed in one-third of the Finnish alcohol poisoning deaths and in over two-thirds of the deaths from alcoholism. The frequency of gastritis was clearly higher in Finland than in the other Nordic countries.

Table 34. Pathological gastric findings among autopsied cases of alcohol poisoning or alcoholism

	Alcohol poisoning				Alcoholism	
Finding	Denmark Per cent	Finland Per cent	Norway Per cent	Sweden[s] Per cent	Finland Per cent	Sweden[s] Per cent
Acute gastritis	8	32	2	13	71	1
Ulcer	—	—	1	2	1	1
Gastric resection	11	5	6	7	6	5
Number of autopsies	61	317	125	238	86	77

Table 35. Statistical significance of the differences in frequency of acute gastritis (p-value)

	Denmark, alcohol poisoning	Finland, alcohol poisoning	Norway, alcohol poisoning	Sweden, alcohol poisoning	Finland, alcoholism
Finland, alcohol poisoning	.000				
Norway, alcohol poisoning	x	.000			
Sweden, alcohol poisoning	.301	.000	.001		
Finland, alcoholism	.000	.000	.000	.000	
Sweden, alcoholism	.048	.000	x	.003	.000

Chi-square contingency test, 1 df

Acute inflammatory changes of the gastric mucosa have been observed in humans after a severe drinking bout (Palmer 1954, 236–238). The lesions caused by alcohol in laboratory animals are the severer the higher the concentration and the larger the volume of alcohol administered (Lorber et al. 1974, 345).

Stress and drugs are other potential causes of gastritis. The importance of stress cannot be assessed, but the effect of drugs seemed to be slight in the present material, since the frequency of gastritis was lower in the Swedish than in the Finnish groups, although drugs had been more commonly resorted to in the former groups.

Alcohol does not influence the frequency of gastric and duodenal ulcer. The same ratio of peptic ulcer has been noted in alcoholics as in the general population (Bingham 1960). In a retrospective follow-up investigation of a group of students, the frequency of peptic ulcer did not correlate with drinking (Paffenbarger et al. 1974). In a cross-sectional study performed on subjects of working age, a U-shaped correlation was found between drinking and peptic ulcer when smoking, which correlated with the frequency of peptic ulcer, was standardized (Friedman et al. 1974). However, investigations on the mortality of alcoholics have shown that the mortality from peptic ulcer is higher in this group than in the general population (Brenner 1967, Schmidt and de Lint 1972). This excessive mortality is probably due to a notable degree to heavy smoking. It appears that drinking as such does not contribute to the development of peptic ulcer. This conclusion is supported by the absence of any clear differences in the present material between the frequency of peptic ulcer and the frequency of gastric resection, notwithstanding the obvious differences in the frequency of gastritis.

Pancreatic findings

Results

Pancreatitis was a rare finding in the present material. This abnormality was somewhat more frequent in the Finnish alcoholism and alcohol poisoning groups than in the other Nordic alcohol poisoning groups (Table 36). Moreover, pancreatitis was slightly more common in those who had died of alcoholism

Table 36. Pathological pancreatic findings among autopsied cases of alcohol poisoning or alcoholism

Finding	Alcohol poisoning				Alcoholism	
	Denmark Per cent	Finland Per cent	Norway Per cent	Sweden S Per cent	Finland Per cent	Sweden S Per cent
Pancreatitis	2	5	1	2	13	5
Fibrosis	2	2	1	1	12	6
Number of autopsies	61	317	125	238	86	77

than in the alcohol poisoning group. Chronic calcifying pancreatitis was observed in three cases in the Finnish alcohol poisoning group and in one case each in the Finnish and Swedish groups of deaths due to alcoholism. The cases of pancreatitis and pancreatic fibrosis were so few that the significance of the differences between the groups was not tested.

Comment

No notable differences in the frequency of pancreatitis were observed between the various Nordic groups of alcohol poisoning deaths. The only group which showed a higher frequency of pancreatitis and pancreatic fibrosis was the Finnish group of deaths from alcoholism. It is noteworthy that chronic calcifying pancreatitis, which is clearly associated with chronic alcohol abuse (Howard and Ehrlich 1961, Sarles and Tiscornia 1974), was present in only about one per cent of the cases, at most.

Previous authors have reported that pancreatitis was observed in about half (Weiner and Tennant 1938, Lundh 1970, Kyösola and Fock 1973) or one-fourth (Ivy and Gibbs 1952) of their series of deaths caused by acute alcohol poisoning (or acute alcoholism). In contrast to these reports, the frequency of pancreatitis was remarkably low in the present material. Since it is known that alcohol is the most common etiological factor for the development of pancreatitis in Swedes (Kager et al. 1972) and in Finnish males (Kyösola and Fock 1973), the impression is obtained that the distinction between acute alcohol poisoning and acute pancreatitis as causes of death is precise in the Nordic countries.

Drug and alcohol poisonings

Results

Among the deaths registered as due to alcohol poisoning, combined drug and alcohol poisonings were clearly most frequent in Sweden, with Denmark in second place (Table 37). Barbiturates and psychopharmaceutics were frequently found in the Swedish cases, barbiturates in the Danish. The most significant differences in drug use were noted between the Swedish group of alcohol poisoning deaths and all other groups and between the Danish alcohol poisoning group and the Finnish groups of deaths caused by alcoholism or alcohol poisoning and the Norwegian group of alcohol poisonings (Table 38).

Psychopharmaceutics were a clearly more common finding in the Swedish alcohol poisoning group than in the other corresponding groups ($p = .000–.030$). The same was found for barbiturates ($p = .000–.011$), with the exception of the difference between the Swedish and the Danish alcohol poisoning deaths (p = .821). Analgesics were notably more often observed in the Swedish alcohol poisoning group than in the corresponding Finnish and Norwegian groups (p = .031–.002).

In the Swedish alcohol poisoning group, drug use was often connected with suicidal tendencies. According to the records, suicidal threats and/or earlier

Table 37. Post-mortem evidence of drug intake among autopsied cases of alcohol poisoning or alcoholism

Drug group	Alcohol poisoning				Alcoholism	
	Denmark	Finland	Norway	Sweden[s]	Finland	Sweden[s]
	Per cent	Per cent	Per cent	Per cent	Per cent	Per cent
Barbiturates	18	3	2	17	–	5
Other soporifics	2	0	–	3	–	1
Psychopharmaceutics	3	4	2	13	–	3
Analgesics	2	3	–	7	1	5
Total	25	10	4	40	1	14
Number of autopsies	61	317	125	238	86	77

Table 38. Statistical significance of the differences in frequency of drugs detected on forensic chemical examination (p-value)

	Denmark, alcohol poisoning	Finland, alcohol poisoning	Norway, alcohol poisoning	Sweden, alcohol poisoning	Finland, alcoholism
Finland, alcohol poisoning	.002				
Norway, alcohol poisoning	.000	.037			
Sweden, alcohol poisoning	.036	.000	.000		
Finland, alcoholism	.000	.007	x	.000	
Sweden, alcoholism	.124	.290	.009	.000	.001

Chi-square contingency test, 1 df

suicidal attempts had occurred in 15 cases (5 per cent) in that group, but rarely in the other groups. In 12 of these 15 cases drugs, chiefly barbiturates and analgesics, were found in the tissues on chemical examination performed at autopsy.

Comment

The proportion of combined drug and alcohol poisonings among the deaths registered as alcohol poisoning was considerably larger in Sweden than in the other Nordic countries. This may be due to a more frequent use of drugs among Swedish heavy users in general, possibly attributable to some special cause, such as a desire for a euphoric experience different from that produced by alcohol, alleviation of anxiety, or attempted suicide. The significance of these factors cannot be evaluated on the basis of the present data.

In spite of the scantiness of information on suicical tendencies produced by police inquiries, such a tendency could be proved in about 5 per cent of the Swedish group of alcohol poisonings, though only in a few cases in the other groups. Moreover, since drug use was clearly more frequent in this Swedish group than in any other group, it seems reasonable to assume that a suicidal tendency explains the high frequency of combined drug and alcohol poisonings in Sweden. This assumption is supported by the fact that among 40 deaths registered as alcohol poisonings in Sweden in 1966, five were later assessed as probable suicides (Berfenstam et al. 1969). The occurrence of concealed suicides among accidental deaths has been attributed to the Swedish classification regulations, which instruct that a probable suicide should be registered as an accidental death, although suicide would in these cases be the proper alternative according to the WHO rules (Berfenstam et al. 1969). Evidence of a similar nature is provided by the fact that the proportion of alcoholics among those who have attempted suicide seems to be larger in Sweden than in the other Nordic countries. In series of hospital patients who had attempted suicide chiefly by means of drugs, the proportion of alcoholics was estimated at 13 per cent (Achté and Ginman 1966) and 15 per cent in Helsinki (Harenko 1968), 10 per cent in Copenhagen (Hove 1953) and 18 per cent in Stockholm (Ettlinger and Flordh 1955).

Combined drug and alcohol poisonings constitute a special problem of classification as to the cause of death, since in many instances death cannot be definitely attributed to either alcohol or the drug as such. It is in fact the synergistic effect of the two substances that is the cause of death. However, the Seventh Revision of the ICD (WHO 1957), which was applied in the Nordic countries until 1968, contained no special category of combined drug and alcohol poisoning. In the Eighth Revision (WHO 1967) then adopted, the classification by nature of injury contains a suitable category, namely, N 979 "Alcohol in combination with specified medicinal agents", but the classification by external cause of death still lacks a specific category for these cases. Of the external causes of death classified by intent, the suicidal class E 950, "Suicide and self-inflicted poisoning by solid or liquid substances" or class E 980 of undetermined cases, "Poisoning by solid or liquid substances undetermined whether accidentally or purposely inflicted", are suitable for deaths caused by the combined effect of alcohol and drugs, but neither definition covers the fact that a specific kind of poisoning due to alcohol and drugs in combination is involved. As regards accidental poisonings, there is no choice other than the undetermined class E 869, "Accidental poisoning by other and unspecified solid and liquid substances", unless accidental alcohol poisoning or drug poisoning in themselves constitute a proper definition of the cause of death. Since the cause-of-death classification by external cause, which is usually applied in the statistics published, contains no suitable category for deaths due to drugs in combination with alcohol, the view of these poisoning cases provided by the official statistics may be inaccurate. This seems to be the case in Sweden. Bearing in mind the lower postmortal blood ethanol concentrations and the higher frequency of drugs observed in the Swedish group of alcohol poisoning deaths compared with the other national groups, it seems possible that a proportion of the Swedish drug and alcohol poisoning cases would have been classified in a special category of combined effects, had this been feasible within the framework of the external cause-of-death classification.

Association of pulmonary and gastric abnormalities with fatty liver

Bronchitis and acute gastritis were more frequent in the Finnish group of alcohol poisonings than in the other Nordic groups. A relationship was assumed to exist between the frequency of these findings and the violent drinking habits of the Finns. This assumption can be more thoroughly tested on the basis of the present material.

Fatty infiltration of the liver has been observed after about a week's consumption of alcohol in daily doses typical of heavy users (cf. p. 103). This abnormality may be due to causes other than alcohol, but in the present material alcohol may be regarded as its main cause. Hence, fatty liver may be regarded as a rough indicator of uncontrolled drinking over a period of many days. If the assumption that alcohol was the cause of bronchitis and gastritis in those who had died of alcohol poisoning is valid, these conditions should be found more often in cases showing fatty infiltration of the liver than in those not showing this abnormality.

Material and methods

The percentage distributions of the different pathological findings in the largest groups, the Swedish and Finnish alcohol poisoning deaths, were compared with each other. The other groups were excluded from comparison owing to the small numbers of autopsies performed. The comparisons were carried out within the countries in question in order to ascertain whether the supposed relationship existed not only in Finland but also in Sweden.

In the study groups, a history of diabetes was obtained in one case in Finland and in two cases in Sweden. In one of the latter cases, the diabetes was mild, and fatty liver was not found at autopsy. No cases of gross obesity or severe malnutrition were recorded.

Results

A clearly higher frequency of bronchitis ($p = .002$) and acute gastritis ($p = .000$) was observed in those Finnish victims of alcohol poisoning in whom fatty infiltration of the liver was observed at autopsy than in those in whom this abnormality was not present (Table 39). In the Swedish material the associations of bronchitis ($p = .100$) and gastritis ($p = .160$) with fatty liver were weaker, but the differences pointed in the same direction as in the Finnish group of alcohol poisonings.

The above associations may be attributable not only to alcohol but also to factors connected with the way of life of heavy users, such as poor hygiene, undernourishment and stress. The significance of these factors cannot be separately evaluated, but a correlation with alcohol consumption at the Skid Row level seems probable. However, no clear association of bronchitis or gastritis with

Table 39. Relationship between the occurrence of fatty liver and pathological pulmonary and gastric findings among autopsied cases of alcohol poisoning

	Finland		Sweden [s]	
	Fatty liver		Fatty liver	
Finding	Absent Per cent	Present Per cent	Absent Per cent	Present Per cent
Bronchitis	38	56	5	12
Pneumonia	4	3	3	3
Acute gastritis	20	41	9	17
Ulcer	—	—	2	3
Gastric resection	5	3	9	4
Number of autopsies	173	133	116	114

alcohol consumption at the Skid Row level was found in the fatty liver group or in the group not showing fatty liver.

In about half the cases investigated (49 per cent of all alcohol poisoning deaths in Finland and 44 per cent in Sweden) no data was available on previous drinking habits. Hence, the above analysis, which was performed using Skid Row alcoholism as an indicator, cannot be applied to the total material. The data does not provide any reasonably useful indicator of the factors related to the way of life. As a rough indicator the place of death was chosen, which is not as specific as drinking at the Skid Row level but which is, on the other hand, applicable to almost all cases contained in the material. The place of death does not of course provide any concise information on the previous social status and environment of the deceased, but it may be assumed that people in a good social position are likely to die at home or in somebody else's home if they succumb to fatal alcohol poisoning; they are not likely to die in a common lodging-house or out of doors. The reverse may be assumed for those representing the lowest stratum of society.

In Finland, the distribution of the place of death was largely the same in the two groups compared (Table 40). The proportion of subjects who had died at home was not notably smaller in the fatty liver group than in the group with normal livers ($p = .271$), and the proportion of outdoor deaths was not smaller in the latter than in the former ($p = .489$).

Table 40. Relationship between the occurrence of fatty liver and place of death among Finnish and Swedish subjects who died of alcohol poisoning

Place of death	Finland		Sweden[s]	
	Fatty liver		Fatty liver	
	Absent Per cent	Present Per cent	Absent Per cent	Present Per cent
At home	36	34	50	45
Somebody else's home	10	7	10	13
Rooming house	2	6	5	5
Public transport means	5	2	3	1
Ambulance on the way to hospital	4	3	3	3
Hospital	2	7	9	6
Custody	4	3	1	5
Outdoors	28	32	12	16
Other places	9	7	7	6
Total	100	101	100	100
Number of cases	171	133	116	114
No information	2	—	—	—

In Sweden, the distribution of the place of death was the same in the group of cases showing fatty liver as in the group with normal liver findings (Table 40). The percentage of subjects who had died at home in the latter group did not appreciably exceed the percentage in the former ($p = .487$), and the percentage of outdoor deaths was not much higher in the fatty liver than in the normal-liver group ($p = .440$).

Comment

In Finland, a strong association was observed between the frequency of fatty infiltration of the liver on one hand and the frequency of bronchitis and acute gastritis on the other. This association was also observed in the Swedish material, although the abnormalities in question were on the whole less frequent. Reports of other potential causes of fatty liver than alcohol were rare. Thus, fatty liver may be regarded as an indicator of uncontrolled drinking over a period of many days in these groups. Assumed concomitants of the way of life of heavy users, frequency of drinking at the Skid Row level and frequency of dying out of doors, had no essential influence on the association observed. Therefore, it seems that the high frequency of bronchitis and acute gastritis among the Finnish victims of fatal alcohol poisoning is due to a great extent to their frequent habit of drinking in excess.

X
ESTIMATES OF THE REAL DIFFERENCES IN MORTALITY FROM ALCOHOL POISONING

For the purposes of this investigation it was important not only to analyse the factors which influence alcohol poisoning mortality, but also to estimate the inter-Nordic differences in the real mortality rates and the deviations of these differences from the statistical ones. For this comparison it was necessary to define criteria for probable deaths by alcohol poisoning.

Methods

The following criteria were chosen for the likelihood that death was caused by alcohol poisoning: (1) a postmortal blood ethanol concentration of at least 3 per mille, (2) absence of suffocating vomit in the lower respiratory tract, (3) absence of drug findings at chemical examination, and (4) absence of pancreatitis.

There were two reasons for choosing a postmortal blood ethanol concentration in excess of 3 per mille as a criterion of probably fatal alcohol poisoning. First, the mean postmortal blood ethanol concentration was nearly 3 per mille in all Nordic groups of alcohol poisoning deaths. Since the distributions of the concentrations were unimodal and relatively symmetric, the mean value is well suited as a mark of distinction between probable and improbable cases. Second, the lowest antemortal concentration considered potentially lethal by earlier authors is about 3 per mille (p. 29).

Those among the deceased who had been suffocated by vomit were excluded from the group of probable alcohol poisoning deaths since the fatal mechanism in these instances was different from that involved in alcohol poisoning, and because it cannot be stated without ambiguity that alcohol was the cause of vomiting. Suffocation by vomit may result from nausea due to causes other than alcohol. In the Swedish group of fatal alcohol poisonings, drugs and suffocating vomit were often found in the same cases. It seems possible that drugs had been at least a contributory cause of vomiting.

Cases in which drugs were detected at postmortal chemical examination were excluded because death may have been caused by the synergistic effect of drugs and alcohol. The data on the Swedish alcohol poisoning deaths shows that suicidal tendencies were more often involved in those cases in which both drugs and alcohol had been ingested than in the pure alcohol poisonings. There seems to be a difference with regard to intent between combined drug and alcohol poisonings and pure alcohol poisonings.

Cases showing acute pancreatitis were not accepted as probable alcohol poisoning deaths because pancreatitis is a highly lethal disease (Kyösola and Fock 1973). Alcohol poisoning which is concurrent with pancreatitis cannot be regarded as the decisive cause of death, unless the blood alcohol concentration is very high.

Applying the above criteria, the percentage of probable alcohol poisoning deaths among the autopsied cases was estimated in the different groups of the material. The number of probable alcohol poisoning cases in the total groups was then estimated on the assumption that the percentage of such cases corresponded to the percentage among the autopsied cases. Furthermore, when the study group consisted of a sample, an estimate was made of the number of probable alcohol poisonings among all deaths that had occurred during the years covered by this study.

Results

The various groups differed considerably from each other with regard to the proportion of probable alcohol poisonings among the autopsied cases (Table 41). This proportion was highest in the Finnish group of alcohol poisoning

Table 41. Probable fatal alcohol poisonings among autopsied cases of certified alcohol poisoning or alcoholism*

	Alcohol poisoning				Alcoholism	
	Denmark Per cent	Finland Per cent	Norway Per cent	Sweden [a] Per cent	Finland Per cent	Sweden [a] Per cent
Probable fatal alcohol poisoning	41	58	55	28	6	19
Number of autopsies	54	305	119	226	64	57

* Probable fatal alcohol poisoning is here defined as a case showing a post-mortem blood ethanol concentration of three per mille or over, no obstructing amount of vomit in the lower respiratory tract, and no drugs on chemical examination.

deaths, but the proportion of probable cases was of almost the same magnitude in the corresponding Norwegian group. The Danish group came in third place. The proportion of probable cases in the Swedish group of alcohol poisonings was small, though larger than in the group of deaths from alcoholism. The Finnish alcoholic group included some cases which were probable alcohol poisoning deaths.

The real alcohol poisoning mortality rates in the different Nordic countries were estimated on the basis of the percentages of probable alcohol poisoning deaths and compared with the statistical mortality rates (Table 42). In the population of 15 years and over mortality was found to decrease from 5 to 1 per one million person-years in Denmark, from 64 to 35 in Finland, from 16 to 5 in Norway and from 10 to 2 per one million person-years in Sweden. As regards the statistical mortality rates for alcoholism and the probable alcohol poisoning cases included in these, it was found that the Finnish group of 16 cases contained 1, and the Swedish group of 27 cases contained 3 probable alcohol poisoning deaths per one million person-years in the population of 15 years and over.

On the assumption that no cases which were in fact alcohol poisonings were included among the deaths classified as being due to alcoholism in the Danish and Norwegian official statistics, it is possible to compare the differences between the statistical and the estimated real alcohol poisoning mortality rates in the Nordic countries. The statistical alcohol poisoning mortality rate for Finland was 400 per cent higher than the figure for Norway, 640 per cent higher than the figure for Sweden, and 1 300 per cent higher than the Danish figure,

Table 42. Statistically recorded and probable alcohol poisoning mortality in the Nordic countries 1967–1971

	Mortality (per one million person-years)*			
	Denmark	Finland	Norway	Sweden
Statistically recorded alcohol poisoning mortality	5	64	16	10
Probable alcohol poisoning mortality included in the above	1	35 e	5	2
Statistically recorded alcoholism mortality	3	16	7	27
Probable alcohol poisoning mortality included in the above	..	1 e	..	3 e

* In the population over 14 years old.

calculated on the population aged 15 years and over. When a summing up was made with regard to the probable cases of alcohol poisoning included in the groups of deaths ascribed to alcohol poisoning and alcoholism in the Finnish and Swedish statistics, and when the mean values for the years 1967–1971 were compared, the estimated real alcohol poisoning mortality rate for Finland was 700 per cent higher than the figures for Norway and Sweden and 3 600 per cent higher than the figure for Denmark.

Comment

The difference found to exist between Finland and the other Nordic countries when the statistical alcohol poisoning mortality rates were compared proved to be somewhat greater still on comparison of the estimated real alcohol poisoning mortality rates. The elimination of the effect of differences in classification practice with regard to alcohol poisoning and alcoholism as causes of death did not cancel out the difference between Finland and the other Nordic countries, when the real alcohol poisoning mortality was estimated by certain criteria of uncomplicated alcohol poisoning. The estimates, however, were rough ones.

The postmortal blood ethanol concentration is not an entirely reliable criterion of fatal alcohol poisoning. A considerable decrease from the maximum concentration may occur (p. 32), if the interval between the point of time when this concentration is reached and death is a lengthy one. Since this interval may vary from less than one hour to over 20 hours (p. 33), it is possible that some patients, whose postmortal blood ethanol concentration was under 3 per mille, in fact died of alcohol poisoning, although the probability that death was due to this cause is slight in the group with concentrations of under 3 per mille. Had a value lower than 3 per mille been chosen to represent the lethal level, a larger number of cases, which were in fact alcohol poisoning deaths, would have been included in the group of probable cases, but at the same time many deaths due to some other cause would have been referred to this group. The number of false positive cases would have increased. Judged by the available data on the lethal level of blood alcohol, the criterion chosen seemed to be the best possible. This is somewhat higher than the criterion of 2.5 per mille used in a previous investigation on the reliability of determinations of fatal alcohol poisonings (Alha and Isotalo 1964).

In the absence of reliable data on the distribution of the interval between the time when the maximum antemortal blood ethanol concentration is reached and the moment of death, it cannot be stated whether the alcohol poisoning mortality rates arrived at in this investigation are underestimates or overestimates. In addition to the decrease in ethanol concentration during the above-mentioned interval, it must be borne in mind that some cases of fatal alcohol poisoning are apparently not thoroughly investigated and thus remain unidentified and unrecorded. It seems probable, therefore, that the present results are underestimates. Since cause-of-death inquiries are more thorough in Finland than in the other Nordic countries, the real differences in alcohol poisoning mortality rates between Finland and the other Nordic countries may be smaller than the estimated ones, though probably not by much. In spite of the obvious sources of error that affect the official statistical alcohol poisoning mortality rates in the Nordic countries, it may, therefore, be concluded that the differences between these rates approximate to real differences in alcohol poisoning mortality between these countries, since the errors balance each other out.

XI
DISCUSSION

Judging by both the official statistical mortality rates and the estimated mortality rates, alcohol poisoning mortality is noticeably higher in Finland than in the other Nordic countries. The comparability of the official data on mortality is somewhat vitiated by the inter-country variation in the thoroughness of cause-of-death inquiries and by differences in diagnostic practice. A considerable number of cases which have been classified in Sweden as deaths caused by alcoholism, would in Finland have been attributed to alcohol poisoning. When uniform criteria for fatal alcohol poisoning were applied to the officially recorded deaths from this cause in the four countries compared, and also to the deaths attributed to alcoholism in Finland and Sweden, death rates for alcohol poisoning (per one million person-years in the population aged 15 years and over) of 36 in Finland, 5 in both Sweden and Norway, and 1 in Denmark were obtained for the years 1967—1971. These figures indicate that the differences between the countries were somewhat greater than those revealed by the official mortality rates for alcohol poisoning.

A positive correlation was observed between the frequency of identified fatal poisonings and the frequency of medicolegal autopsies in Finland. This observation together with the ratios of medicolegally autopsied cases to all deaths seems to justify the conclusion that the estimated mortality rates give a somewhat, though probably slightly, exaggerated view of the real inter-country differences. By and large, the real differences in alcohol poisoning mortality between the Nordic countries correspond fairly closely to the statistical differences.

The higher postmortal blood ethanol concentrations observed in the Finnish group of alcohol poisonings seem to constitute evidence of heavier acute intoxication compared with the other national groups. Furthermore, chronic uncontrolled drinking seems to be more common in Finland than in the other Nordic countries. This is indicated by the greater proportion of Skid Row alcoholics in the Finnish group of alcohol poisonings. The fact that bronchitis and acute gastritis, diseases etiologically related to heavy alcohol consumption, were more often found among the Finnish autopsied cases of fatal alcohol poisoning, constitute corroborative evidence of the chronic nature of the violent Finnish drinking habits. The covariation of the frequency of fatty liver and the frequency of bronchitis and acute gastritis shows that the latter diseases are alcohol-related. It can, therefore, be stated that uncontrolled drinking habits seem to constitute the main determinant of the differences in alcohol poisoning mortality between the Nordic countries.

Comparability of alcohol poisoning mortality rates

The data relating to mortality from alcohol poisoning is influenced both by the thoroughness of cause-of-death inquiries and diagnostic practice. The effect of these factors should always be taken into account when the differences in alcohol poisoning mortality between different areas and their causes are subject to investigation.

The thoroughness of cause-of-death inquiries affects the number of detected alcohol poisoning deaths, but the magnitude of this effect is not readily assessed. As regards the differences between the Nordic countries, the effect does not seem to be great.

Data on the circumstances preceding death and on circumstances that may contribute to the fatal outcome is usually scanty unless autopsy has been performed. In the absence of autopsy results the reliability of cause-of-death determinations is low. If autopsy, including chemical examinations, has been performed, a correct diagnosis of alcohol poisoning is more likely. It may be assumed that the number of correctly diagnosed fatal alcohol poisonings increases with the increase in the number of autopsied cases; at the same time there is a decrease in the number of cases which would have been falsely diagnosed as alcohol poisonings without autopsy. In other words, with increasing thoroughness of cause-of-death inquiries the reliability of cause-of-death determinations increases, but this does not necessarily imply that the number of detected alcohol poisoning deaths increases to any considerable extent beyond the number recorded without thorough inquiries.

The above conclusions seem to indicate that the relationship between thoroughness of cause-of-death inquiries and the number of detected fatal alcohol poisonings cannot be expressed by any universally applicable formula. When the effect of thoroughness of cause-of-death inquiries is evaluated, it is always necessary to take into account the different national factors which operate in the countries compared.

Cases which were to be regarded as fatal alcohol poisonings on the criteria selected were found in the Swedish group of deaths attributed to alcoholism and also, though in smaller number, in the corresponding Finnish group. Alcoholism appears to be the cause-of-death category most likely to include cases which are in fact alcohol poisoning deaths. In inter-country comparisons special attention should, therefore, be paid to this group, as well as to other possible diagnostic differences. It is important to clarify the question as to whether alcoholism is used as a diagnostic synonym for alcohol poisoning, or whether definite criteria exist by means of which these two cause-of-death categories can be distinguished. It is also possible that alcoholism is arbitrarily indicated as the underlying cause of death in cases in which other, potentially lethal abnormalities are present (Bruun et al. 1975, 20). If this is so, alcoholism apparently serves as a kind of litter-bin, into which alcohol-related cases difficult to classify are thrown. Alcohol poisonings in which premortal elimination of blood ethanol has led to a considerable drop in the concentration are liable to classification as death by alcoholism. If there is reason to assume that the two cause-of-death categories alcohol poisoning and alcoholism consist of fundamentally similar cases, and if it is not possible to subject the individual cases to close analysis, it seems advisable to combine these groups in inter-country comparisons. It should be borne in mind, however, that this does not guarantee comparability, since both groups may include erroneously diagnosed cases, the proportion of which may vary from country to country.

The Swedish groups of deaths caused by alcohol poisoning and alcoholism contained cases in which suicidal tendencies were demonstrable and in which both alcohol and drugs were detected on chemical examination. It has been stated that the Swedish instructions on coding by cause of death favour a classification as accidental poisoning in cases which in fact should be regarded as suicides (Berfenstam et al. 1969). Moreover, it has been assumed that suicidal poisonings in Sweden are also concealed in the group of undetermined fatal poisonings (Beskow 1974, Kastengren 1974). The Swedish suicidal poisoning mortality rates are, therefore, not directly comparable with the corresponding figures for the other Nordic countries. In inter-country comparisons special attention should be directed to the erroneous classification of combined drug and alcohol poisoning suicides as accidental or undetermined poisonings.

In cases of combined drug and alcohol poisoning, death is often caused by the synergistic effect of alcohol and drugs, rather than by the alcohol effect or the drug effect as such. Classification of these cases by the external cause of death is difficult when the death is accidental, since the E classification of causes of accidental deaths includes no special category for combined poisonings. A choice has to be made between accidental alcohol poisoning (E 860) and accidental poisoning by drugs and medicaments (E 850—859). If combined poisonings tend to be differently classified in different countries, the results of comparisons will be biased. For this reason cause-of-death statistics should also be published according to the N classification, which contains a special class for combined poisonings (N 979). Furthermore, a corresponding class in the E classification may be recommended for introduction in the next revision of the ICD.

Criteria of fatal alcohol poisoning

Fatal alcohol poisoning is not accompanied by any typical patho-anatomical changes. The ethanol concentration in the blood is the most reliable, although not an infallible, criterion for the distinction between alcohol poisoning and other possible causes of death.

The average lethal ethanol concentration in the blood seems to be about 5 per mille. This represents the maximum concentration reached during intoxication. However, the maximum blood ethanol level has seldom been determined in fatal cases. As a rule, the question as to whether death was caused by alcohol poisoning must be decided on the basis of the postmortal blood ethanol concentration, which approximates very closely to the concentration prevailing at the moment of death. This is usually lower than the maximum concentration, since the blood ethanol concentration falls during the interval between the time when the maximum concentration is reached and the moment of death. This interval varies greatly from a few minutes to as much as 24 hours. On the basis of the relevant literature (p. 33), the interval may be estimated at an average of seven hours. The rate of disappearance of ethanol from the blood during this period varies from about 0.16 to 0.41 per mille per hour (p. 35) in heavy drinkers and alcoholics, who constitute the group most likely to fall victims to fatal alcohol poisoning. The weighted average* for the blood ethanol decline rates (p. 34) recorded in eight studies comprising a total of 134 observations of the decline rate in alcoholics was 0.258 per mille per hour. According to these premises, the average fall of blood ethanol from the peak value to the concentration prevailing at the moment of death would be 1.8 per mille, and the average postmortal blood ethanol concentration in victims of fatal alcohol poisoning would be 3.2 per mille. Incidentally, this is approximately the same value as that chosen on other grounds as a criterion for probable fatal alcohol poisoning when attempting to assess the real alcohol poisoning mortality rate (p. 113).

If the length of the interval between the maximum blood ethanol concentration and the moment of death were known, it would be possible to estimate the peak value more precisely. However, even then the individual variation in blood ethanol decline rate, which is considerable, would remain a source of uncertain-

* The sum of the means for the study groups multiplied by the weights, i.e. the ratio of the number of cases in the study groups to the number of all observations.

ty in the calculations. There also seems to be a noticeable individual variation in the lethal level of blood alcohol, since a concentration of as little as 3 per mille has been considered potentially lethal and yet it has been reported that intoxicated persons have survived concentrations exceeding 7 per mille. Thus, the diagnosis of fatal alcohol poisoning is in general a probabilistic, not a deterministic, decision.

How drinking leads to fatal alcohol poisoning

The conclusion that chronic uncontrolled drinking is the factor responsible for the variations in alcohol poisoning mortality is more tenable if the underlying process leading to a lethal concentration of ethanol is understood. There are two possible mechanisms: (1) an increase in the blood ethanol concentration resulting from increasing tolerance and (2) an accumulation of ethanol in the organism over long periods of drinking.

As physiological tolerance develops, the capacity of the organism to compensate the functional impairment caused by alcohol increases (Kalant 1973). A steadily rising blood ethanol concentration is, therefore, required to produce the same functional impairment that resulted from previous drinking bouts. Since functional impairment seems to be a prerequisite of euphoria, it may be assumed that it is necessary for drinkers to take steadily larger doses in order to attain the desired effect. If it is true that tolerance does not develop to the lethal alcohol concentration (Koppanyi et al. 1961), the blood alcohol concentration required for the desired euphoric experience apparently approaches increasingly closer to the lethal level as drinking continues. However, the question as to whether tolerance to the lethal effect does or does not develop is still an open one.

The other mechanism enhancing the risk of fatal alcohol poisoning is the accumulation of ethanol in the organism. During excessive drinking bouts the alcohol ingested may exceed the amount which the organism is capable of eliminating. It has been estimated that Swedish liver cirrhosis patients consume up to 355 grams ethanol daily (Hällén and Krook 1963). One sixth of the Danish alcoholics interviewed in 1965–1967, representing the heaviest drinkers, had a median daily consumption of about 420 grams of 100 per cent ethanol (Diderichsen and Skyum-Nielsen 1969, 115). In a Finnish investigation it was estimated that alcoholics of no fixed abode in the town of Tampere in 1970–1971 consumed about 470 grams ethanol in the summer and about 380 grams in the winter per ordinary drinking day (Murto 1972, 177). On the assumption that the maximum rate of elimination of ethanol is about 0.2 grams per kg of body weight per hour (Lelbach 1974, 102–104) and that the average body weight is about 70 kg, it may be estimated that the organism is capable of eliminating an average of 336 grams ethanol daily, at most. During a period of uncontrolled drinking the amount of ethanol ingested in some instances exceeds the eliminating capacity of the organism, and the result is an accumulation of alcohol. With continued drinking the blood alcohol concentration also rises, and the risk of fatal alcohol poisoning increases.

Both the mechanisms described above seem to be relevant from the standpoint of arriving at an understanding of how chronic uncontrolled drinking leads to death. The observations that the peak in the age distribution of the victims of fatal alcohol poisoning in the Nordic countries fell in the age group 45—54, that death was frequently preceded by long periods of drinking, and that the mortality rates for public holidays were not exceptionally high, seem to indicate that the deaths caused by alcohol poisoning, although classified as accidental, are usually not random results of occasional, violent drinking. To a great extent the risk of fatal alcohol poisoning should be predictable and death preventable.

Distinction of alcohol poisoning as a cause of death

The typical victim of severe alcohol use ending in death is the middle-aged chronic alcoholic, who dies suddenly, without revealing any prior symptoms of disease. The findings made at post-mortem examination are often fatty infiltration of the liver and elevated blood ethanol concentration. In these cases it is often possible to choose between three different underlying causes of death: alcoholism, alcohol poisoning and liver cirrhosis. All three alternatives are resorted to.

The varying diagnostic usage with regard to alcohol-related deaths is amply exemplified in the literature. In North Carolina (Fatteh and Hayes 1974, McBay and Hudson 1974) and Texas (Costello and Schneider 1974), alcohol poisoning is often indicated as the cause of death when this has been preceded by alcohol consumption. In New York City corresponding cases are classified as deaths from alcoholism, the criterion usually being an alcohol concentration of 3 per mille or more in the blood or brain tissue. Even if no alcohol can be demonstrated in the tissues of the deceased, acute alcoholism may be considered as the cause of death if this has been preceded by unconsciousness or hospital treatment (Haberman and Baden 1974). Chronic alcoholism is diagnosed on the basis of abnormalities resulting from long-standing alcohol use. These are fatty infiltration and cirrhosis of the liver, jaundice and liver failure, bleeding oesophageal ulcers and ascites. A series of deaths classified as caused by liver cirrhosis in Baltimore, Maryland, included some sudden deaths in which fatty liver without any changes indicative of cirrhosis were found; in some cases the postmortal blood alcohol concentration exceeded 1.5 per mille (Kramer et al. 1968). In a study from Florida, about 30 per cent of sudden unexpected deaths from disease related to complications of alcohol use were considered to have been caused by alcoholic fatty liver (Davis 1975).

The similarity between alcoholism and liver cirrhosis is brought forward in an investigation dealing with mortality in 12 American cities. When the mortality rates for alcohol psychosis and alcoholism were combined, Guatemala City ranked first in mortality with a figure of 529 per one million person-years calculated on the male population aged 15—74 years (Puffer and Griffith 1967, 161—163). On analysing the deaths from alcoholism in Guatemala City the authors found that 45 out of 118 cases showed either obvious cirrhosis or fatty infiltration of the liver. They stated in conclusion: "Some of these deaths, had they occurred elsewhere, might have been attributed to cirrhosis rather than to chronic alcoholism." (Puffer and Griffith 1967, 163).

The variation in diagnostic usage shows that the death of a chronic alcoholic, when it occurs in a state of intoxication, is not always readily explained. At the same time, as regards the origin of this interpretational variability the question arises: is it due to the nature of the statutes governing the determination of cause of death or to conceptual differences?

Deaths are statistically recorded according to the underlying cause of death. This is "(a) the disease or injury which initiated the train of morbid events leading directly to death, or (b) the circumstances of the accident or violence which produced the fatal injury" (WHO 1967, 469). The question of whether alcohol poisoning, alcoholism or cirrhosis of the liver should be indicated as the cause of death relates to causality, as evidence of all these conditions is often found in one and the same case.

In a situation when the choice of the underlying cause of death may be made between two alternatives, alcoholism and alcohol poisoning, the chronologically acceptable causal order implies that alcoholism be considered the underlying cause of death, precipitating the immediate cause of death, which is alcohol poisoning. However, the regulations on the determination of the cause of death contain two points which argue against this interpretation: (1) Alcoholism as a disease category is less specific than alcohol poisoning; according to the *rule of specificity* (WHO 1967, 424), alcohol poisoning is therefore preferable as an underlying cause of death. Moreover (2), the WHO rules do not state that alcoholism as a cause-of-death category involves alcohol poisoning (WHO 1967, 149).

In alcohol-related deaths, liver cirrhosis is a rare finding, while fatty infiltration of the liver is frequently observed. According to the rules of WHO, classification by liver cirrhosis (571.0) as the underlying cause of death may then be indicated, as fatty infiltration of the liver is included in this category

(WHO 1967, 219). When fatty liver presents itself as a diagnostic alternative beside alcoholism and alcohol poisoning, a possible permutation is that (chronic) alcohol poisoning or alcoholism be considered as the underlying cause of death and fatty infiltration of the liver as the immediate cause of death, resulting from the former. However, this solution is invalidated by (1) the rule of specificity and (2) the rule of codification which says that if alcoholism occurs as an underlying cause of death in connection with liver cirrhosis, the two causes of death should be combined so that alcoholic liver cirrhosis is indicated as the underlying cause of death (WHO 1967, 219 and 427). This rule also applies to cases in which liver cirrhosis or fatty infiltration is considered as the underlying cause of death and alcoholism as a contributory cause.

The above discussion relates to a situation in which three causes of death — alcohol poisoning, alcoholism and cirrhosis of the liver — have to be considered and the point at issue is their integration in a way that complies both with the rules of causality and with the codification rules of the WHO. The principles discussed above do not apply of course if only one cause of death is relevant in the opinion of the medicolegal expert investigating the case or — with regard to coding — if only one cause has been indicated in the death certificate.

Other possible alternatives for alcohol poisoning (E 860) as the cause-of-death category are the categories of suicide by solid or liquid substances (E 950), deaths by solid or liquid substances undetermined as to whether self-inflicted or accidental (E 980), and homicide (E 962). One problem is the definition of intent of the activity connected with alcohol poisoning. However, alcohol-related poisoning which is not accidental seems to be very rare (Harenko 1968). When the documents were revised, no suicides were judged to have taken place among 117 cases that had officially been classified as death from accidental alcohol poisoning in Helsinki in 1960—1961 and 1970—1971 (Lönnqvist 1977, 41). In an investigation of deaths by poisoning that occurred in England and Wales in 1968—1970, among 85 alcohol poisonings two were considered to be suicides and 83 accidental (Barraclough 1974).

The group of indeterminate deaths, in which the question of intent remains open, may conceal alcohol poisonings. This is exemplified by nine cases coded as indeterminate, which the National Institute of Forenisic Medicine in Lund considered to be alcohol poisonings. Deaths caused by the combined effects of drugs and alcohol may easily be coded as indeterminate, since the classification by external cause (E classification) contains no group of accidental deaths which seems quite appropriate for combined poisonings (p. 120).

A comparison of alcohol poisoning, alcoholism and liver cirrhosis as alternative causes of death should include consideration of whether the alternative chosen can lead to death by any known mechanism. Where this is not the case, the alternative in question cannot be considered the *cause* of death. If it is possible to choose another cause of death, which is associated with a clearly lethal mechanism, this is to be preferred.

The choice between different diagnoses is also a question of conceptual differences. As a medical concept, alcoholism is less well-defined than alcohol poisoning. Jellinek (1960, 36—38) stated that there are several "alcoholisms" and that some of them are not morbid conditions; they are either cultural habits (beta alcoholism) or a means of relieving pain (alpha alcoholism). Jellinek only classified drinking from a compulsive inner need (gamma and delta alcoholism) as really morbid. However, the compulsive nature of drinking cannot be assessed by any known criteria, and it cannot be proved that a need to drink oneself to death is involved.

As a concept, alcohol poisoning is more appropriate than alcoholism in medical science, bearing in mind that the acute and chronic effects of substances that are deleterious to the organism are generally called poisoning. In point of fact alcoholism was apparently originally a synonym for alcohol poisoning. Magnus Huss (1807—1890), generally regarded as the man who invented the term alcoholism, stated: "Den sjukdom, hvilken förekommer hos sådana, som missbrukat alkoholhaltiga drycker och som ofvan blifvit skildrad under benämningen Alcoholismus chronicus, öfverensstämmer med chroniska förgiftningssjukdomar i allmänhet." ("The disease occurring in persons who have abused alcoholic beverages and which is described above under the name of Alcoholismus chronicus corresponds to poisonous diseases in general.") (Huss 1849, 191). Only since the distinction of alcohol poisoning as an alternative diagnosis has alcoholism become a separate concept, and one which confuses the analysis of alcohol-related problems more than it contributes to their clarification. Use of this term has produced a fallacy, namely, that the lethal effect of an exogenous poison is regarded as a death from natural causes.

XII
SUMMARY

Mortality from alcohol poisoning was markedly higher in Finland than in Denmark, Norway and Sweden during the period 1961–1973. The causes of the differences were analysed on the basis of official statistical data, statutes relating to inquiries into the cause of death, and medicolegal records of deaths from alcohol poisoning and alcoholism. It was assumed that differences in the degree of thoroughness in tracing the cause of death, in diagnostic practice in establishing the cause of death and in drinking habits would explain the differences observed in mortality from alcohol poisoning. It was considered likely that a diagnosis of alcoholism was sometimes used as an alternative for one of alcohol poisoning.

This investigation utilizes the official statistical data on alcohol poisoning and alcoholism mortality for the years 1961–1973. The body of the material consists of six groups, for which data was collected from death certificates and autopsy records, mainly from the years 1967–1971. In the four alcohol poisoning groups there were 106 cases in Denmark, 328 cases in Finland, 238 cases in Norway and 325 cases in Sweden. The number of cases in the two alcoholism groups was 118 for Finland and 115 for Sweden. The alcoholism groups and the Finnish alcohol poisoning group were drawn as systematic samples, while the remaining groups included all deaths that occurred during the study period.

Differences and trends in statistically recorded mortality

The consistency and significance of the differences in mortality were assessed by analysing both the official statistical data by age and sex groups and the trends in mortality. In males, the mortality rate from alcohol poisoning in Finland was 93, in Norway 22, in Sweden 15 and in Denmark 6 per million person-years in 1967–1971. The mortality from alcoholism in Sweden was 38, in Finland 23, in Norway 10 and in Denmark 4 per million person-years. All inter-country differences in mortality in males were significant. Age standardization somewhat enhanced the inter-country differences in mortality from alcohol poisoning and reduced the differences in mortality from alcoholism. Most of the inter-Nordic differences in mortality from alcohol poisoning were due to the differences in male mortality, the female mortality rates being markedly lower than the rates for males. The inter-country differences in mortality from alcohol poisoning and alcoholism in females paralleled the differences in males.

The peak in age-specific mortality from alcohol poisoning occurred in Finland and in Norway in the age group 45—49, while the peak was observed in Sweden in the age group 50—54. The highest age-specific mortality rates from alcoholism were observed in Finland in the age group 45—49, in Norway in the age group 65—69 and in Sweden in the age group 50—59. The age-specific alcohol poisoning mortality was higher even in the Finnish males aged only 25—29 years than in any age group of Danish or Swedish males, and the mortality in Finnish males aged 30—34 years exceeded the highest Norwegian figure.

The five-year moving averages for the age-standardized mortality rates showed that mortality from alcohol poisoning increased in all the Nordic countries and in both sexes during the period 1961—1973 except in Danish males. The increase was greatest in Finland. Mortality from alcoholism also increased in all the Nordic countries during the same period, the greatest increase occurring among Swedish and Finnish males.

Differences in mortality between provinces

The variation in mortality from alcohol poisoning and alcoholism between different provinces was analysed, because the occurrence of factors explaining mortality was assumed to correlate with population density and level of development of the regions in question. Alcohol poisoning mortality in Norway was greatest in the most developed region, Oslo, while in Finland it was greatest in the most sparsely populated provinces, i.e. Lapland, Central Finland and Oulu. In Sweden no noticeable variation in mortality from alcohol poisoning was observed between the various provinces. Mortality from alcoholism was concentrated in the most densely populated areas, the province of Stockholm in Sweden and the province of Uusimaa in Finland. No deaths from alcohol poisoning occurred in the province of Åland, which is the part of Finland closest to Sweden both geographically, linguistically and culturally. The concentration in densely populated and urbanized regions implied that the quantity of alcohol consumed together with social rootlessness are of importance as causative factors. On the other hand, the fact that mortality from alcohol poisoning was high in sparsely populated provinces in Finland and low in the province of Åland suggested that culturally determined drinking habits are a notable cause of alcohol poisoning mortality.

Thoroughness in inquiring into the causes of death

The thoroughness in inquiring into the causes of deaths was assumed to influence the number of deaths from alcohol poisoning actually recorded in the different Nordic countries. The proportion of deaths in which medicolegal autopsy was performed, calculated on the total number of deaths, was considered a rough indicator of thoroughness. During the period 1967–1971 this proportion was 13 per cent in Finland, 7 per cent in Sweden, 2 per cent in Denmark and about 1 per cent in Norway. The differences between the countries were easily understandable when one compares the statutes concerned with obligatory investigation of the cause of death.

There was greater scope under Finnish and Swedish law for cause-of-death examinations on the suspicion of death from poisoning than was the case under Danish and Norwegian laws. In Finland and Sweden physicians were obliged to inform the police of suspected deaths by poisoning. In Denmark and Norway this obligation only applied when foul play was suspected. In these countries it was within the province of the police to order a medicolegal examination to be performed only on the suspicion of foul play, while in Finland and Sweden the law also made it possible for the police to demand an investigation on the suspicion of poisoning. In Finland, physicians were not authorized to write a death certificate without being sure of the cause of death. Swedish physicians had the right to refuse to write a certificate in such cases, while in Denmark and Norway physicians were obliged to issue a death certificate even when the police had not ordered an autopsy.

The relationship between the thoroughness of cause-of-death examinations and statistically recorded mortality was estimated by determining the correlation between the number of medicolegal autopsies and the number of accidental deaths by poisoning in 12 Finnish provinces during the period 1963–1971. The correlation coefficient (+.48) was highly significant. According to variance interpretation the number of autopsies accounted for about 23 per cent of the variation in mortality. Together, the correlation observed and the differences between the Nordic countries as regards the extent of possible inquiries, differences which are legal in nature, show that thoroughness is a significant factor in explaining mortality from alcohol poisoning.

Diagnostic differences

It seemed likely that alcoholism and alcohol poisoning in Sweden were used as alternative diagnoses, while in Finland these conditions were regarded as diagnostically different categories. To substantiate this, the males in Finland and Sweden whose death was attributed to alcoholism were compared to those who had died of alcohol poisoning. In Finland, persons who died of alcoholism were more often Skid Row alcoholics, suffering more often from fatty liver and pancreatitis, and their postmortal blood ethanol concentration was lower than in the group who died of alcohol poisoning. In Sweden, the two groups did not differ significantly with regard to these factors. The comparison showed that alcohol poisoning and alcoholism were regarded as separate entities in Finland, while these diagnoses were used as alternatives in Sweden. A diagnosis of alcoholism was preferably used at the National Institute of Forensic Medicine in Stockholm, while alcohol poisoning was preferred as a diagnosis at the other institutes.

The classification of those cases which in Finland were considered as deaths from alcohol poisoning into other cause-of-death categories in the other Nordic countries was studied by comparing the frequency of pathological findings in the males whose death was attributed to alcohol poisoning to the statistical death rates for certain causes of death in 1967–1971. No differences were observed which could be interpreted as evidence for the assumption that a large number of deaths from alcohol poisoning were concealed in the groups in which alcohol psychosis, acute or indeterminate bronchitis, liver cirrhosis, acute pancreatitis, senile marasmus, sudden death (cause unknown), freezing, drowning, aspiration of gastric contents or suicidal poisoning was judged to be the cause of death. The results showed that no notable differences due to the classification of causes of death occurred, except that the diagnoses of alcoholism and alcohol poisoning ran parallel in Sweden.

Implications of the differences in drinking habits

The significance of differences in drinking habits was estimated by analysing certain phenomena related to death from alcohol poisoning, which were considered as indicators of the intensity and frequency of uncontrolled drinking in the different Nordic countries. Deaths occurred in Finland on Midsummer Day, in Sweden on the first of May and on Midsummer Day more often than could be attributed to chance. Despite the statistical significance of the differences, the concentration of deaths on these holidays was slight. The postmortal blood ethanol concentration in those who had died of alcohol poisoning in Finland was 3.2, in Norway 3.0, in Sweden 2.6 and in Denmark 2.6 per mille. The proportion of drinkers at the Skid Row level in Finland was 38 per cent, in Norway 25 per cent, in Denmark 22 per cent and in Sweden 13 per cent. Industrial alcohol substitutes leading to death at one drinking bout were more often used and the number of deaths that occurred out of doors was larger in Finland than in the other Nordic countries. The rate of mortality from alcoholism was 17 per million person-years among Swedish citizens of Swedish origin, while the corresponding figure for the Finnish immigrants in Sweden was 112 per million person-years. These results indicate that a large proportion of those who had died from alcohol poisoning were chronic drinkers, whose alcohol consumption was distributed over many days, but nonetheless culminated to some extent on special holidays. The intoxication of those dying from alcohol poisoning seemed to be greater and the number of Skid Row alcoholics and users of industrial alcohol substitutes seemed to be larger in Finland than in the other Nordic countries. The tradition of uncontrolled drinking seemed to be borne out among the Finnish immigrants in Sweden by their considerably higher mortality from alcoholism, compared to the Swedes, a mortality which may be attributed to alcohol poisoning, bearing in mind the differences in diagnostic practice discussed above.

Pathological findings

Heavy drinking was assumed to influence the frequency of pathological findings in the deceased. The victims of fatal alcohol poisoning in Denmark, Finland, Norway and Sweden and those who had died of alcoholism in Finland and Sweden were therefore compared with regard to the frequency of pathological findings. Bronchitis was more common in Finland among those who had died of alcohol poisoning (46 per cent) and alcoholism (45 per cent) than in any other group (6—21 per cent). Suffocation by aspiration of gastric contents had occurred more often in Sweden among those dying from alcoholism (19 per cent) and alcohol poisoning (17 per cent) than in any other group (7—9 per cent). Of cardiac abnormalities, myofibrosis was more frequent among the Swedes who had died of alcohol poisoning (36 per cent) than in any of the other groups (3—22 per cent); myocardosis was discovered only in those Finns who had died of alcoholism (26 per cent) or alcohol poisoning (8 per cent). Fatty liver was observed among those who had died of alcohol poisoning in 51 per cent in Denmark, in 49 per cent in Sweden, in 43 per cent in Finland and in 42 per cent in Norway. Among those whose death was attributed to alcoholism, fatty liver was found in 85 per cent in Finland and in 56 per cent in Sweden. Acute gastritis was clearly more common among the Finnish victims of alcoholism (71 per cent) and alcohol poisoning (32 per cent) than in the other groups (1–13 per cent). Similarly, pancreatitis was more frequently observed among Finns who had died of alcoholism (13 per cent) than in any other group (1–5 per cent). Bronchitis, gastritis, fatty liver and pancreatitis are conditions which have a strong etiological association with alcohol use. The higher frequency of bronchitis and gastritis among the Finns compared to the other Nordic countries seemed, therefore, to be to a great extent attributable to the level of consumption.

When chemical analyses were performed in connection with autopsy, drugs – usually barbiturates or psychopharmaceutics – were most frequently detected in the Swedish victims of alcohol poisoning (39 per cent), with the Danish alcohol-poisoned in second place (25 per cent), while the figures for the remaining groups were much lower (1–14 per cent). In Sweden, suicidal tendencies had been noticed in a large proportion of those who had died of alcohol and drug poisoning. Considering that among those who had attempted suicide with the aid of drugs, the proportion of alcoholics appeared to be greater in Sweden than in the other Nordic countries, the conclusion may be drawn that among those constituting a suicidal risk group the simultaneous use of drugs and alcohol as a means of relieving anxiety is perhaps most common in Sweden.

Since fatty liver may be considered an indicator of heavy alcohol consumption over several days, the association of bronchitis and gastritis with fatty liver was determined in order to assess more precisely the significance of the level of alcohol consumption. The significance of way of life was estimated by comparing the frequency of pathological findings in Skid Row alcoholics and in those who had died out of doors with the frequency in other cases of alcohol poisoning in Finland and Sweden. Bronchitis and gastritis were found to be more common among those who had fatty liver than among those in whom this condition was not observed. In contrast, no significant relationship was noticed between alcohol consumption at the Skid Row level or dying out of doors and the presence of fatty liver. The conclusion was drawn that the variation in frequency of bronchitis and gastritis depended mainly on the quantity of alcohol consumed.

Estimated real differences in mortality

To estimate the real differences in mortality from alcohol poisoning, those cases were selected which fulfilled the following criteria of death as being probably due to alcohol poisoning: postmortal blood ethanol concentration three per mille or more, absence of a suffocating amount of aspirated gastric contents, absence of pancreatitis and absence of postmortally detected drugs. These criteria were applied to those who had died of alcohol poisoning in all the Nordic countries and to those who had died of alcoholism in Sweden and Finland. When alcohol poisoning mortality rates were calculated on the basis of the cases thus selected, the inter-country differences turned out to be somewhat greater than the statistical differences. On the other hand, had the level of investigation been the same in all countries, the differences would probably have been smaller than the statistical differences. Hence it may be established that, despite the sources of error inherent in the official statistical data, the view of the inter-country differences in mortality from alcohol poisoning obtained from them is remarkably accurate, since the errors balance each other out.

To sum up, it may be stated that (1) differences in thoroughness in inquiring into the causes of deaths explain the inter-country differences in mortality, though clearly only to some extent, (2) the low mortality from alcohol poisoning in Sweden is in part due to the fact that a proportion of the cases are diagnosed as deaths from alcoholism, (3) the inter-country differences are mainly attributable to variations in the frequency of uncontrolled alcohol consumption, aimed at producing a state of deep intoxication, and (4) that the inter-country differences as estimated on the basis of the official statistical data on alcohol poisoning mortality are of the same magnitude as the real differences, despite the sources of error inherent in the statistics.

APPENDICES

APPENDIX 1

ORGANIZATION OF MEDICOLEGAL CAUSE-OF-DEATH INQUIRIES IN THE NORDIC COUNTRIES

This appendix presents in broad outline the statutes relating to cause-of-death inquiries and the organization and activities of the medicolegal services in the different Nordic countries in 1966–1971. The aim is to pick out those features which affected the identification of alcohol poisoning deaths in these countries during the period covered by this investigation.

Denmark

Statutes

Ligsynsloven, the Danish Act of January 2, 1871, relating to the examination of dead bodies, forbids burial of the body before it has been examined and a death certificate issued. The examination is primarily the duty of the physician who attended the deceased person during his or her last illness. If the physician in question has a lawful excuse for not examining the body, or if the deceased person has not been attended by a physician, it usually falls to a local medical officer to undertake the examination. If the medical officer is prevented from doing this, any physician living in the place where the death in question occurred is duty bound to perform the task. If the domicile of the nearest physician is farther away than two kilometres, two special inspectors *(Ligsynsmænd)* may be called in. These are appointed by the Chief Constable on the recommendation of the parish council (Gormsen 1973, 77–78).

The question of when a medicolegal, and when a medical, inquiry into the cause of death should be made is settled by the *Ligsynsloven* which states in 6 §:

"Opstår der ved ligsynet formodning om, at dødsårsagen fortjener justitsvæsenets opmærksomhed, skal lægen, ligsynsmændene eller jordemoderen uopholdeligt gøre indberetning herom til politimesteren, og dødsattest må da ikke udstedes, førend denne har tilkendegivet, at der fra hans side intet er til hinder herfor.

(If on examination of the dead body a suspicion arises that the cause of death is worth the attention of the judicial system, it is the duty of the physician, the inspectors of the dead body or the midwife to report this to the Chief Constable immediately, and a death certificate must not be issued until the latter has stated that he has no objections to this.)"

This paragraph has been interpreted as implying that physicians are duty bound to inform the police (1) when a person has been found dead, (2) when death has resulted from an accident, suicide or homicide, (3) when death has been preceded by an accident, suicidal attempt or attempted homicide, and (4) when it seems possible that some other person has caused the death (Gormsen 1973, 82). However, physicians are not obliged to report a sudden, unexpected death to the police.

In Denmark the police decide whether a medicolegal cause-of-death inquiry be carried out. The practical application of this rule is based on its interpretation by the Ministry of Justice as put forward in a letter of May 23, 1921. If the police do not consider a medicolegal inspection of the dead body or autopsy warranted, physicians are obliged to write an ordinary death certificate even against their own convictions (Gormsen 1973, 82). The police should order a medicolegal autopsy (1) if it is known or suspected that foul play is connected with the death, (2) if there is reason to assume that a suspicion of foul play can arise later, and (3) if it is thought possible that death was caused by some other person's criminal negligence (Gormsen 1973, 101). Apart from the medicolegal autopsy, the police may order a "police autopsy". This is done if it is assumed that the case will not be subject to the processes of law, but clarification of the cause of death is deemed desirable in order to eliminate suspicion. This may be the case if death has been sudden and unexpected and the cause unknown. The relatives of the deceased cannot refuse an autopsy ordered by the police (Gormsen 1973, 102).

The police are not obliged to order a medicolegal cause-of-death inquiry in all cases reported to them. The above-mentioned letter by the Ministry of Justice of May 23, 1921, states that the police may refrain from ordering a medicolegal autopsy when the deceased person has not been found dead, or when the case is not of sufficient interest from their standpoint (Gormsen 1973, 122). Hence, in Denmark accidental deaths are not subject to medicolegal investigation (Gormsen 1973, 83).

The physician who examines the body notes in the death certificate the underlying cause of death, the class of death and data relating to operations and autopsy, if performed. If the inspection is medicolegal, a police inquiry is made.

The circumstances preceding death, the circumstances relating to the death and the observations made on examination of the body should also be noted in the death certificate (Gormsen 1973, 83—84). Even though autopsy is performed, it is not mandatory to make any notes on the findings in the death certificate, which may be sent to the registry before the autopsy report has been written. The National Health Service of Denmark is in charge of the cause-of-death statistics, and this authority also determines what is to be recorded as the underlying cause of death. If it appears from the death certificate that autopsy has been carried out, although the findings have not been noted down at the point reserved for this purpose, the National Health Service orders an inquiry and the underlying cause of death is determined on receipt of the findings (Hamtoft 1973, personal communication).

Structure

There are some 63 medical officers *(Embedslæger)* in charge of the medicolegal examinations of dead bodies. There are 14 provincial medical officers *(Amtslæger),* 46 district medical officers *(Kredslæger),* the municipal medical officer of Copenhagen and the provincial medical officers of the Faroes and Greenland. The medical officers carry out medicolegal examinations of dead bodies, sign the death certificates issued on the basis of medicolegal cause-of-death inquiries and attend at medicolegal autopsies when necessary. Medicolegal autopsies (including "police autopsies") are carried out by special legal pathologists *(Statsobducenter),* appointed by the State and active at the University Institutes of Forensic Medicine in Copenhagen and in Odense and at the Department of Forensic Medicine in Aarhus (Gormsen 1973, 10—11). Forensic chemical examinations are performed at the University Institute of Forensic Medicine in Copenhagen, at the Department of Forensic Medicine in Aarhus and at the Pharmacological Department, University of Copenhagen (Gormsen 1973, 103).

Activities

The majority of autopsies carried out in Denmark are medical. During the period covered by this investigation, medical autopsy was performed in about 42 per cent of all deaths, while medicolegal autopsy was performed in only about 2 per cent (Table 43). The low frequency of medicolegal autopsies is counterbalanced by the relatively high frequency of medicolegal external inspections: 9 per cent during the period in question.

Medicolegal post-mortem blood alcohol determinations have been performed at the University Institute of Forensic Medicine in Copenhagen and,

Table 43. Cause-of-death inquiries in Denmark 1967–1971

Year	Medicolegal		Medical	Total number of deaths
	Autopsies	External post-mortems	autopsies	
	Per cent	Per cent	Per cent	
1967	2.3	8.5	40.2	47 836
1968	2.3	9.0	41.7	47 290
1969	2.3	9.2	42.6	47 943
1970	2.4	9.4	43.1	48 233
1971	2.5	9.6	43.5	48 858
Total	2.4	9.1	42.1	240 160

since 1968, also at the Department of Forensic Medicine of Aarhus University. The total number of post-mortem blood alcohol determinations was 1 111 in 1966 and 1 457 in 1971. During the period 1966–1971, blood alcohol determinations were performed on an average of 3 per cent of all deceased persons.

Finland

Statutes

During the period 1967–1971, medicolegal cause-of-death inquiries were carried out as stated in 8 § of the statute of 1889 on the enforcement of the Criminal Code and as stated in the modification of this statute by an Act of 1959 (192/1959). As regards the basic rules for medicolegal inquiries the law states:

"Jos joku tavataan kuolleena eikä tiedetä hänen tautiin kuolleen tai jos joku muutoin on kuollut sellaisissa olosuhteissa, jotka osoittavat tai antavat aihetta epäillä, että hän on omasta tai toisen kädestä saanut surmansa, on poliisin heti suoritettava asiassa tutkinta, tarvittaessa käyttäen lääkäriä apunaan. Jollei kuoleman syytä varmuudella voida todeta ulkonaisen ruumiintarkastuksen perusteella, on asianomaisen poliisipiirin päällikön ratkaistava, onko asiassa toimitettava oikeuslääkeopillinen ruumiinavaus ennen kuin kuolleen saa haudata.

(If a person is found dead and disease is not known to be the cause of death, or if a person has otherwise died under circumstances which indicate or give rise to the suspicion that he has been killed by his own or somebody else's hand, it is the duty of the police to inquire immediately into the case, and if necessary to summon expert medical assistance. If the cause of death cannot be established with certainty by external inspection of the body, it is the duty of the Chief of the police district in question to decide whether a medicolegal autopsy should be carried out before burial of the body be permitted.)"

8 § of the statute on the enforcement of the Criminal Code implies that a cause-of-death inquiry should be performed (1) if a person is found dead and it is not certain that he or she has died of natural causes, or (2) if there is suspicion of foul play. This paragraph seems to imply that the police conduct an inquiry and a physician examines the dead body. If the cause of death is not then established with certainty, the Chief of police is authorized to decide whether a medicolegal autopsy be performed.

Medicolegal external inspection of the dead body is performed by a physician summoned by the police to assist in the cause-of-death inquiry. Medical officers are obliged to perform this task, but the police may invite some other physician who is willing to assist. If the physician finds that he can identify the cause of death with certainty on the basis of external inspection, he can issue a death certificate. In their general instructions on medicolegal cause-of-death investigations, the National Board of Health stated (April 8, 1947) that a death certificate must not be issued unless the cause of death is completely clear. It is further specified that external inspection of the body is sufficient only if the data on the case fulfils the need for information required for a death certificate.

Furthermore, if a person has died in hospital, but with violence or poisoning as possible contributory causes of death, a medicolegal cause-of-death inquiry is considered necessary. The instructions issued by the National Board of Health to hospital physicians (February 27, 1964) state that this category includes unforeseen deaths and deaths suspected or known to be caused by accident, suicide or poisoning. The Finnish laws and regulations imply that a medicolegal cause-of-death inquiry be performed if alcohol poisoning is suspected to be the cause of death, and that autopsy including forensic chemical examinations be carried out if it cannot be stated without ambiguity that alcohol poisoning is the only demonstrable cause of death. However, owing to a certain lack of precision in the wording of 8 § of the statute on the enforcement of the Criminal Code, these measures are not always adopted. There has been some disagreement between the medical profession and the police concerning the interpretation of this paragraph. The sentence "If a person is found dead and disease is not known to be the cause of death," has been interpreted by physicians as meaning that all unexpected deaths as well as deaths caused by accident, suicide or poisoning should be subject to medicolegal autopsy. The police, on the other hand, consider a medicolegal autopsy necessary only in cases in which there is a suspicion of foul play (Oikeuslääketieteellisten... 1971, 74–75). The fact that the police interpret this paragraph more narrowly than the medical profession and that the police are in a position to decide whether medicolegal autopsy be performed or not may in some cases be responsible for inadequate examination of alcohol poisoning deaths and erroneous definition of the cause of death.

There has been some debate concerning the rules relating to the death certificate. According to the statute on medicolegal cause-of-death inquiries, physicians have the right to refuse to issue a death certificate, but according to the rules relating to death certificates a medical officer is obliged to write a death certificate, even though he was not the last doctor to attend the deceased person (Oikeuslääketieteellisten... 1971, 76). If a physician refuses to issue a death certificate, it does not follow that autopsy is automatically performed. The Chief of police makes the final decision.

Structure

During the period 1967–1971, the Finnish provincial medical officers carried out medicolegal autopsies. In 1969, autopsies were performed by 12 provincial medical officers and five assistant provincial medical officers. In Helsinki, medicolegal autopsies were performed at the Helsinki University Department of Forensic Medicine. Medicolegal autopsies on persons who died in or near Turku were carried out at the Department of Forensic Medicine of Turku University. In the Department of Forensic Medicine at the University of Oulu medicolegal autopsies were carried out on persons who died in the province of Oulu.

The specimens taken at autopsy were examined microscopically at the Departments of Forensic Medicine of the Universities of Helsinki, Turku and Oulu. Forensic chemical examinations were usually performed at the Division of Forensic Chemistry of the Helsinki University Department of Forensic Medicine.

In Finland, forensic chemical examinations are only performed on cases subject to medicolegal cause-of-death investigation (Oikeuslääketieteellisten... 1971, 90–91). Statute 172/1947 stipulates that medicolegal autopsy should be carried out within eight days from the day on which the order was received from the police, that the autopsy report should be sent to the provincial government within eight days from autopsy, and that the provincial government should forward the report to the National Board of Health within eight days.

Activities

During the period 1967–1971, autopsy was performed in about 31 per cent of all deaths in Finland (Table 44). Medicolegal autopsy was performed in 13 per cent and medical autopsy in 17. 5 per cent. Determination of the cause of death

Table 44. Cause-of-death inquiries in Finland 1967–1971

Year	Medicolegal		Medical		Total number of deaths
	Autopsies	External post-mortems	Autopsies	External post-mortems	
	Per cent	Per cent	Per cent	Per cent	
1967	11.5	.3	15.4	2.8	43 790
1968	11.6	.3	16.4	3.8	45 013
1969	13.2	.2	17.5	2.9	45 776
1970	13.7	.2	18.9	2.3	43 986
1971	14.9	.1	19.3	3.7	45 752
Total	13.0	.2	17.5	3.1	224 317

was based on external inspection of the body in only about 3 per cent of all deaths. In about 66 per cent of cases the cause of death was recorded in accordance with the diagnosis made on examination and treatment of the deceased person during his or her last illness. The proportion of both medicolegal and medical autopsies increased steadily during the study period. The ratio of medicolegal autopsies rose during this time by about 30 per cent.

Medicolegal post-mortem blood alcohol determinations were performed in a total number of 1 554 cases in 1967 and 1 524 in 1968 (Alha 1970b, 382 and 387). Most of these were performed at the Division of Forensic Chemistry, Helsinki University Department of Forensic Medicine, the remainder at the Department of Forensic Medicine, Turku University. Determination of blood alcohol was performed in about 3 per cent of all deaths.

Norway

Statutes

In Norway, the relatives or spouse of a deceased person are obliged to report the death as stipulated in § 12 of the Act of 1930. In cities and towns the report is sent to the court of distribution *(skiftesretten),* in rural districts to the bailiff *(lensmannen).* If there are no close relatives to report the death, this task is incumbent upon other persons who are well-informed about the case. In some instances, particularly if there is a suspicion of suicide or homicide, a physician summoned to the place may report the death. The death report may be made either (1) verbally by two adult persons who have seen the deceased after death has occurred or (2) by the issuing of a death certificate (Lundevall 1973, 45).

Physicians are duty bound to issue a death certificate if they have been present at the moment of death or if they have seen the dead body. It is not necessary for the physician to know the cause of death when he writes the death certificate. A physician is not authorized to issue a death certificate without having seen the dead body first, and physicians are not obliged to inspect the body. A physician who inspects the dead body may either sign or refuse to sign the following clause in the death certificate:

> ”Undertegnede lege erklærer herved at det ikke er grunn til å anta at døden er voldt ved en straffbar handling.
> (The undersigned physician declares that there is no reason to suspect that death is due to foul play.)”

Even if a physician is unwilling to append his name to this clause, he is not duty bound to report the case to the police. On the other hand, physicians are obliged to notify the police where a death is not due to natural causes and where it may be assumed that foul play is involved (263 § of the Act of 1887 on the processes of law in criminal cases). Notification is primarily the duty of the relatives of the deceased person, but the paragraph in question has been interpreted as implying that physicians are duty bound to inform the police if suspicion arises of a relative or relatives of the deceased person being involved in foul play (Lundevall 1973, 45—46). Norwegian physicians are faced with a very difficult task in cases where they have to distinguish between the possiblity of foul play and deaths which may be due to natural causes. If there is suspicion of foul play, a medicolegal investigation should be performed as stipulated in 211 § of the Act of 1887 on the processes of law in criminal cases (Lundevall 1973, 21). This paragraph delegates to the police the power to order medicolegal cause-of-death inquiries and to decide the form they will take (Lundevall 1973, 46).

The duty of notifying the police is also mentioned in two other laws. 5 § of the Act of 1898 on post-mortem procedures stipulates that the transportation of a dead body abroad is forbidden without the permission of the police. If foul plaly is suspected or if it cannot be stated with certainty that death was due to natural causes, permission is withheld by the police until an appropriate medicolegal investigation has been performed. 4 § of the Act of 1913 on cremation stipulates that the local police are authorized to grant permission for cremation on the same conditions that apply to the transportation abroad of a dead body. A prerequisite for permission by the police in these cases is that a medical officer *(embedslege)* who has inspected the dead body writes a certificate in which the cause of death is indicated and it is stated whether foul play is suspected or not. A similar certificate is also required from the physician who attended the deceased person during his or her last illness (Lundevall 1973, 45—46).

When dealing with an application for cremation, the police in Norway are compelled to ascertain the cause of death and decide whether a medicolegal investigation is required. The situation is similar when permission is sought to transport a dead body abroad. On the other hand, if the deceased person's relatives prefer inhumation, the police are only obliged to consider the question of cause-of-death investigation if this is warranted by information received from the relatives or a physician. The restriction on the physician's authority to notify the police in cases of this kind implies a source of uncertainty and error as regards cause-of-death statistics. Lundevall (1973, 47) assumed that a proportion of homicides and deaths caused by another person's actions or criminal negligence in Norway escapes the notice of the police.

Structure

Outside hospitals and nursing homes, cause-of-death investigations are mainly performed by medical officers *(offentlige leger),* either provincial medical officers *(fylkesleger)* or district medical officers *(distriktleger).* In towns, any physician is authorized to inspect a dead body. In rural districts a death certificate may be issued by the bailiff, who notes down what the relatives of the deceased person consider to be the cause of death. The death certificate is sent to a medical officer, who forwards it to the Central Bureau of Statistics of Norway. When the police have ordered a medicolegal cause-of-death investigation, the death certificate is usually signed by the medical officer who inspected the dead body. The medical officer may be a medicolegal expert.

Medicolegal autopsies are performed at the Institute of Forensic Medicine of Oslo University, the Department of Pathology of Bergen University and the departments of pathology of the major hospitals. The autopsy report and the cause of death as established on the basis of this report are not always available when the death certificate is signed and sent to the Central Bureau of Statistics. If a death certificate is officially stamped by the Institute of Forensic Medicine or one of the departments of pathology, or if the death certificate indicates that autopsy has been performed, the officials at the Central Bureau of Statistics procure additional data by means of a questionnaire or by a personal visit to the archives of the Institute or the department in question. If additional data is obtained, the statement on the cause of death is usually altered in accordance with the autopsy result (Lettenstrøm 1973, personal communication).

Activities

The autopsy ratio is very low in Norway. During the study period 1967–1971 only about 12 per cent of all deceased persons were autopsied (Table 45). Medicolegal and medical autopsies are not distinguished in the official

Table 45. Cause-of-death inquiries in Norway 1967–1971

Year	Autopsy	Treatment or examin- ation during last illness	External post-mortem and earlier treatment or examination	No earlier treatment	Total number of deaths
	Per cent	Per cent	Per cent	Per cent	
1967	11.7	76.1	1.9	10.3	36 216
1968	11.5	77.0	1.2	10.3	37 668
1969	12.0	76.6	1.7	9.7	38 994
1970	12.7	75.6	1.4	10.3	38 723
1971	12.4	76.8	1.5	9.3	38 981
Total	12.1	76.4	1.5	10.0	190 582

Norwegian statistics. It is known, however, that during the years 1966–1969 the number of medicolegal autopsies ranged between 315 and 371 (Oikeuslääketieteellisten... 1971, 24). It may, therefore, be assumed that during the study period about 1 per cent of all deaths were subjected to medicolegal autopsy and about 11 per cent to medical autopsy. Furthermore, it seems probable that the ratio of medicolegal autopsies to all deaths did not appreciably exceed 2 per cent. According to the law, copies of all reports on investigations in criminal cases requiring medicolegal expert knowledge should be sent to a medicolegal commission *(Den rettsmedisinske kommisjon)* set up in 1900 (Lundevall 1973, 25). During the period 1967–1971 this commission received an average of 880 reports annually. On the assumption that all reports deal with medicolegal autopsies, the ratio of these to all deaths would be about 2.3 per cent. However, a proportion of the reports dealt with external inspections of dead bodies or forensic psychiatric examinations.

During the study period the majority of deceased persons in Norway were not subjected to any thorough post-mortem examination. In 76 per cent of cases a death certificate was issued on the basis of examination performed and/or treatment given during the deceased person's last illness (Table 45). Ten per cent had apparently not received any treatment.

Post-mortem blood alcohol determinations in Norway are performed by Oslo University Institute of Forensic Medicine and the National Institute of Forensic Chemistry. No data was obtained on the number of alcohol determinations performed at the former institute; the latter performed a total of 460 determinations in 1968–1971, or an annual average of 115.

Sweden

Statutes

In Sweden a physician is obliged to issue a death certificate if the deceased person was under the physician's care during his or her last illness, if mother or child died during delivery conducted by the physician, or if the physician inspected the body after death. If a physician finds that he cannot write a death certificate on the basis of what is known about the deceased person's last illness or on the basis of inspection of the dead body, further investigations should be carried out (Socialstyrelsen 1971, 11–12).

A physician is considered to have been in charge of a deceased person during his or her last illness if care was a lengthy process. The physician is authorized to issue a death certificate only if it is probable that the illness in question was the cause of death. If the patient was under the physician's care only for a short time or care was limited to certain therapeutic measures, the physician is considered to have performed therapeutic measures but not to have been in a position to perform examinations which would warrant a definite stand with regard to the disease that caused death. In this case it cannot be stated that the physician was in charge of the patient, and the obligation to write a death certificate does not, therefore, apply. Inspection of the dead body is considered sufficient grounds for issuing a death certificate if it was thorough enough to permit establishment of the probable cause of death. A physician who has only performed an external inspection of the body and finds further examinations desirable is not obliged to write a death certificate (Socialstyrelsen 1971, 12–13).

The Swedish law and its interpretation, therefore, presuppose that thorough information is available or that further examinations are performed before a death certificate is issued.

If a physician cannot write a death certificate on the basis of the available data, the police should immediately be informed about the case. This obligation applies when the physician has not performed the examinations necessary for the establishment of the cause of death, or when the examinations performed have revealed that further clarification is required. This is the case for instance when disease is not the only cause of death. Moreover, deaths should always be reported to the police (1) when the identity of the deceased person is unknown, (2) when there is reason to suspect that death is not due to disease alone, (3) when the results of a cause-of-death inquiry can help to disclose a crime which may be indirectly connected with the death, and (4) when the results of a cause-of-death inquiry can clear somebody of suspicion of criminal involvement. These stipulations apply to deaths occurring outside hospitals.

Deaths occurring in hospitals and nursing homes should be reported to the police (1) if the identity of the deceased person is unknown, (2) if it is assumed that medicolegal autopsy is required, and (3) if the findings made at medical autopsy suggest that the death has been caused by others or that suicide is involved. These instructions have been interpreted as implying that when there is anything to suggest that a death is not due to disease alone, or when the time of treatment has been too short to permit thorough clinical examinations, the physician should consider reporting the case to the police unless the possibility of foul play can be completely ruled out. Deaths caused by poisoning, injury and assault and battery belong to this category. In uncertain cases it is preferable to notify the police, after which it is the obligation of the police to decide about the need for further investigation (Socialstyrelsen 1971, 16).

On notification by a physician about the need for a cause-of-death inquiry, the police in Sweden decide on the measures to be adopted. The police should perform without delay a preliminary investigation, the principal aim of which is to clarify whether foul play is involved or not (Socialstyrelsen 1971, 17). According to the law, the decision on medicolegal investigations is taken by a court of law, the provincial government, the public prosecutor or the Chief of police. The authority who decides that a medicolegal autopsy be performed is obliged to hand over to the medicolegal expert an account of their proceedings and other documents which may be of help in performing the investigation (Socialstyrelsen 1971, 8). Instead of a medicolegal autopsy, the police may order a complete cause-of-death investigation *(fullständig dödsorsaksundersökning)* or a simple cause-of-death investigation *(enkel dödsorsaksundersökning)*. No binding instructions, only suggestions, have been issued on the choice of method of investigation. A physician who has been requested by the police to perform a medicolegal investigation of a certain type may direct an application to the responsible authority that a more thorough investigation be performed.

The most exacting medicolegal investigation, medicolegal autopsy, is resorted to when death is or may be due to foul play. A medicolegal autopsy is justified when the possibility of foul play cannot be ruled out. A complete cause-of-death investigation is a less thorough autopsy, which is mainly used in the examination of injuries sustained in road accidents as well as for fatal poisonings. In the latter cases, forensic chemical examination for alcohol and other poisons is recommended. If neither of the above-mentioned types of autopsy seems to be required, a simple cause-of-death investigation may be performed, the aim of which is mainly to establish the probable cause of death (Socialstyrelsen 1971, 18—19). The main difference between medicolegal autopsy and a complete cause-of-death investigation is that the former can only be performed by a specialist and a copy of the autopsy report has to be sent to the Council of Medicolegal Experts *(Rättsläkarrådet)*. A simple cause-of-death investigation differs from a complete cause-of-death investigation in that no autopsy report is required and the scope of the examination may be limited to the establishment of the probable cause of death (Saldeen s.d.).

Structure

In Sweden it is mainly the duty of medicolegal experts to perform medicolegal cause-of-death investigations. Autopsies are performed at the national institutes of forensic medicine in Gothenburg, Lund, Stockholm, Umeå and Uppsala. Each medicolegal institute has its area of responsibility, which comprises three to six provinces. Since medicolegal autopsies can be performed only at these five institutes, transportation may be a lengthy process and the waiting time protracted. For this reason physicians other than medicolegal experts are entrusted with simple cause-of-death investigations. Investigations of this kind are, for instance, delegated to physicians working at the departments of pathology of certain hospitals (Socialstyrelsen 1971, 17).

Activities

The autopsy ratio calculated on all deaths was high in Sweden during the study period: 7 per cent for medicolegal, 39 per cent for medical and 46 per cent for all autopsies (Table 46). External inspection of the dead body was an infrequent form of cause-of-death investigation. The ratio of both medicolegal and medical autopsies increased from 1967 to 1971, the ratio of medicolegal autopsies by as much as 74 per cent.

Postmortal blood alcohol determinations were performed at the National Institute of Forensic Chemistry, Stockholm. No statistical data was obtainable on the number of alcohol determinations performed during the study period. In 1972, chemical analyses were performed in connection with 3 509 autopsies (Jakobsson 1973).

Table 46. Cause-of-death inquiries in Sweden 1967–1971

Year	Autopsy		Examination before death		External post-mortem	Total number of deaths
	Medicolegal	Other	Death in hospital	Death somewhere else		
	Per cent	Per cent	Per cent	Per cent	Per cent	
1967	5.7	38.6	37.6	12.0	4.5	78 994
1968	6.2	39.2	38.1	11.1	3.9	81 767
1969	7.5	39.0	38.5	9.2	3.9	83 306
1970	7.6	39.4	40.2	7.9	3.6	80 023
1971	9.9	39.1	39.9	6.3	4.3	82 734
Total	7.4	39.1	38.9	9.3	4.1	406 824

APPENDIX 2

VALIDITY OF POSTMORTAL BLOOD ETHANOL CONCENTRATION

After death changes are known to occur which result in the formation of ethanol in the body (pp. 35–37). If alcohol has been consumed, the value obtained at ethanol determination performed post mortem may be higher than the concentration prevailing at the moment of death, owing to postmortal ethanol formation. The question may, therefore, be posed as to whether the values for ethanol obtained from blood drawn at autopsy are valid measures of the ethanol concentration at the time of death.

It may be assumed that the formation of ethanol post mortem is larger in proportion to the length of the time lapse from death to the collection of blood samples. In the Nordic countries blood specimens are almost invariably obtained at autopsy. Hence, it may be assumed that the longer the interval between death and autopsy, the higher the ethanol concentrations observed, provided postmortal ethanol formation has any notable effect on the blood ethanol level. Since the dichromate method reacts not only to ethanol but also to other volatile organic substances, it may be assumed that higher values for blood ethanol are obtained by this method than by the enzymatic or gas chromatographic methods, provided the changes occurring post mortem are considerable and the interval between death and autopsy is lengthy.

The effect of the postmortal ethanol formation was assessed by cross-tabulating the blood ethanol concentration and the interval between death and autopsy, utilizing the available data on the total Nordic material of deaths from alcohol poisoning and alcoholism. Statistical significance was determined by the chi-square contingency test. Time was classified in accordance with the experimental results of Wolthers (1958).

The association between the postmortal blood ethanol concentration measured by the enzymatic or gas chromatographic methods and the inverval between death and autopsy was not significant ($p = .820$). The mean ethanol concentration was practically the same in all time-classes (Table 47). The blood ethanol concentration measured by the dichromate method increased slightly as time interval from death became longer (Table 48). However, there was no

Table 47. Post-mortem blood ethanol concentration measured by an enzymatic or gas chromatographic method at various times after death

Blood ethanol concentration (per mille)	Time after death (days)		
	Less than three	Three to four	Over four
–0.99	23	17	13
1.00–1.99	54	39	35
2.00–2.99	103	71	55
3.00–3.99	145	95	92
4.00–4.99	35	24	16
5.00–	1	3	4
Total	361	249	215
Arithmetic mean of blood ethanol concentration (per mille)	2.78	2.79	2.79

Table 48. Post-mortem blood ethanol concentration measured by the dichromate method at various times after death

Blood ethanol concentration (per mille)	Time after death (days)		
	Less than three	Three to four	Over four
–0.99	11	8	3
1.00–1.99	12	17	15
2.00–2.99	35	31	30
3.00–3.99	50	47	68
4.00–4.99	27	26	17
5.00–	1	1	5
Total	136	130	138
Arithmetic mean of blood ethanol concentration (per mille)	3.02	3.07	3.17

strong association between concentration and time ($p = .071$). The slight increase of the concentrations may well be attributable to the fact that the dichromate method also reacts to other volatile organic substances, in contrast to the enzymatic and gas chromatographic methods.

It may be concluded that the postmortal ethanol formation did not influence the blood ethanol concentration to any noteworthy extent in the material studied. The postmortal blood ethanol values measured by an enzymatic or gas chromatographic method may, therefore, be considered as valid measures of the concentration at the time of death.

ACKNOWLEDGEMENTS

This investigation, performed in 1972–1977, was sponsored chiefly by the Finnish Foundation for Alcohol Studies (Research Director: Docent Kettil Bruun, Ph. D.), which placed funds and technical facilities at my disposal. The final extent of the investigation was an outcome of the stimulating atmosphere at my place of work, the Department of Public Health Science, University of Helsinki (Director: Professor Ilari Rantasalo, M.D.). Some of the results were analysed while I was working at the Department of Public Health, University of Tampere (Director: Professor Mauri Isokoski, M.D.). I am deeply indebted to the Directors of these institutions for their encouragement and support.

Close Scandinavian contacts were a prerequisite for my work. These were mediated by the Northern Committee for Alcohol Research. During the period of planning and acquisition of material, many people in the various Scandinavian countries generously sacrificed their time in offering me both intellectual and practical assistance. My gratitude is due to all of them for their helpfulness and valuable suggestions. I wish particularly to mention the following persons:

In Denmark: Professor Jørgen B. Dalgaard, M.D., the Department of Forensic Medicine, University of Aarhus, Professor Harald Gormsen, M.D., Dr. Alf Lund, Ph.D., and Dr. Jørgen Voigt, M.D., the University Institute of Forensic Medicine, Copenhagen, Mr. H. Hamtoft, the National Health Service of Denmark, Copenhagen, Chief Physician Egill Jensen, M.D., the Forchhammersvej Outpatient Department of the Copenhagen Hospital Services, Dr. Svend Juul, M.D., the Institute of Social Medicine, University of Aarhus, Chief Physician Andrej Myschetzky, M.D., Bispebjerg Hospital, Copenhagen, Dr. Johannes Nielsen, M.D., University Institute of Psychiatry, Aarhus, and Professor Jørn Simonsen, M.D., the University Institute of Forensic Medicine, Odense.

In Finland: Professor Antti Alha, M.D., the Division of Forensic Chemistry, Department of Forensic Medicine, University of Helsinki, Chief of Forensic Office Antti Isotalo, M.D., National Board of Health, Helsinki, and Statistician Aino Korpela, M.A., Central Statistical Office of Finland, Helsinki.

In Norway: Chief Physician Per Anchersen, M.D., Ullevål Hospital, Oslo, Dr. Sverre Brun-Gulbrandsen, Pol.Sc.D., the National Institute for Alcohol Research, Oslo, Ms. Ragnhild Bækken and Ms. Lita Holan, the Central Bureau of Statistics of Norway, Oslo, Professor Jon Lundevall, M.D., and Dr. Jens Hognestad, M.D., the Institute of Forensic Medicine, University of Oslo, and Professor Per Sundby, the Institute of Social Medicine, University of Oslo.

In Sweden: Emeritus Professor Carl Henry Alström, M.D., Bureau Chief Anne-Marie Bolander, M.D. (hon.), the National Central Bureau of Statistics, Stockholm, Professor Roger Bonnichsen, M.D., the National Institute of Forensic Chemistry, Stockholm, Dr. Kerstin Boström, M.D., the National Institute of Forensic Medicine, Gothenburg, Dr. Bertil Falconer, M.D., and Dr. Sten V. Jakobsson, M.D., the National Institute of Forensic Medicine, Stockholm, Professor Leonard Goldberg, M.D., and Docent Ulf S. Rydberg, M.D., the Department of Alcohol Research, the Karolinska Institute, Stockholm, Emeritus Professor Gunnar A.R. Lundquist, Professor Tom Saldeen, M.D., the National Institute of Forensic Medicine, Uppsala, Dr. Milan Valverius, M.D., the National Institute of Forensic Medicine, Umeå, and Professor Gerhard Voigt, M.D., the National Institute of Forensic Medicine, Lund.

It would not have been possible to collect the material without the favourable attitude adopted by various authorities in the Nordic countries towards this study. I am indebted to the National Health Service of Denmark, the Finnish Ministry for Social Affairs and Health, the Norwegian National Board of Health, the Swedish National Board of Social Welfare, and the Heads of the 27 Swedish hospitals who kindly allowed me to utilize the records relevant to my investigation.

I am grateful for stimulating discussions with the following research workers at the Finnish Foundation for Alcohol Studies and the Social Research Institute of Alcohol Studies: Dr. Salme Ahlström-Laakso, Pol.Sc.D., Mr. Eero Lahelma, M.Pol.Sc., Docent Klaus Mäkelä, Pol.Sc.D., Mr. Juha Partanen, Lic.Pol.Sc., Mr. Pekka Sulkunen, M.Pol.Sc., Ms. Sirkka-Liisa Säilä, M.Pol.Sc., and Mr. Esa Österberg, M.Pol.Sc. I also wish to thank the personnel at the Library and Information Service of the State Alcohol Monopoly of Finland, in particular Mr. Jarmo Heinonen, M.Pol.Sc., and Mr. Erkki J. Immonen, Lic.Pol.Sc., for their help in procuring the literature I needed for my work.

Professor Antti Alha, M.D., Docent Kettil Bruun, Ph.D., Docent Mikko Salaspuro, M.D., Professor Kai Sievers, M.D., and Professor Henrik Wallgren, Ph.D., all from the University of Helsinki, devoted many strenuous hours to the perusal and discussion of consecutive versions of my manuscript. Their constructive criticism was invaluable, and I wish to express my deep gratitude and appreciation to all of them.

My gratitude for assistance in applying the statistical methods is due in particular to Associate Professor Seppo Sarna, Ph.D., the Department of Public Health Science, University of Helsinki, and Mr. Jussi Simpura, M.Sc., the Social Research Institute of Alcohol Studies, Helsinki. The views put forward by Professor Olli S. Miettinen, M.D., Ph.D., School of Public Health, Harvard University, U.S.A., on the epidemiological methods and concepts have influenced the presentation of the results.

Ms. Eva Palmgren, M.A., acquainted herself thoroughly with the theme of my work, translating it into fluent and readable English. The translation was checked by Mr. Peter Jones, B.A. My thanks are due to both of them.

Ms. Leila Iivonen and Ms. Eeva-Liisa Tuovinen drew the diagrams. Ms. Tuula Muhonen checked the manuscript for printing. Ms. Anja Lepo, B.M., M.Sc., and Ms. Leena Tuominen, M.Sc., helped me in the choice of programs for data processing. Mr. Juhani Turunen solved the problems connected with the data processing swiftly and skilfully. I am indebted to all the above-mentioned persons and other members of the personnel at the Department of Public Health Science, University of Helsinki, and the Social Research Institute of Alcohol Studies, for the help they have given me.

This investigation is published simultaneously in the series edited by the Finnish Foundation for Alcohol Studies (Volume 28) and in the series Alcohol Research in the Northern Countries. The publication in the latter series was financially supported by the Scandinavian countries via the Northern Committee for Alcohol Research.

Kari Poikolainen

REFERENCES

ACHTÉ, K. A. & GINMAN, L.: Suicidal attempts with narcotics and poisons. *Acta Psychiatr. Scand.* 42:214–232, 1966.

AHLSTRÖM-LAAKSO, SALME: *Drinking habits among alcoholics*. The Finnish Foundation for Alcohol Studies, vol. 21, Forssa 1975.

AHMED, S. SULTAN; LEVINSON, GILBERT E. & REGAN, TIMOTHY J.: Depression of myocardial contractility with low doses of ethanol in normal man. *Circulation* 48:378–385, 1973.

ALHA, A. R.: *Blood alcohol and clinical inebriation in Finnish men. A medico-legal study*. Ann. Acad. Sci. Fenn. (Med.) No. 26, Helsinki 1951.

ALHA, ANTTI: Alkoholi ja oikeuslääketiede (Alcohol and forensic medicine). *Alkoholikysymys* 42:3–30, 1974.

ALHA, ANTTI: Alkoholi ja sydänlöydökset vuonna 1967 oikeuskemiallisesti tutkituissa kuolemantapauksissa (Alcohol and heart findings among forensic-chemically investigated cases of death in 1967). *Alkoholikysymys* 38:3–12, 1970a.

ALHA, ANTTI: Oikeuskemian yleisosa (General part of forensic chemistry). Pp. 381–404 in *Oikeuslääketiede* (Forensic medicine), ed. Unto Uotila. WSOY, Porvoo 1970b.

ALHA, ANTTI & ISOTALO, ANTTI: *On acute fatal poisonings in Finland in 1958 and their detection*. Ann. Med. Exp. Biol. Fenn. 42: Suppl. 1, 1964.

ALLARDT, ERIK: *Att ha, att vara, att älska – Om välfärd i Norden* (Having, being, loving – On welfare in the Nordic countries). Argos förlag AB, Kalmar 1975.

ALLARDYCE, D. BRUCE: The postmortem interval as a factor in fat embolism. *Arch. Pathol.* 92:248–253, 1971.

ALSTRÖM, C. H.; LINDELIUS, ROLF & SALUM, INNA: Mortality among homeless men. *Br. J. Addict.* 70:245–252, 1975.

ANDRÉASSON, RUNE & BONNICHSEN, ROGER: Resultat av klinisk undersökning vid olika alkoholhalter (Results of clinical examinations at different alcohol concentrations). *Alkoholfrågan* 58:204–207, 1964.

ARKY, RONALD A.: The effect of alcohol on carbohydrate metabolism: carbohydrate metabolism in alcoholics. Pp. 197–227 in *The biology of alcoholism,* volume 1; *Biochemistry,* eds. Benjamin Kissin & Henry Begleiter. Plenum Press, New York 1971.

ARKY, RONALD & FREINKEL, NORBERT: Hypoglycemic action of alcohol. Pp. 67–80 in *Biochemical and clinical aspects of alcohol metabolism,* ed. V. M. Sardesai. Charles C. Thomas, Springfield, Ill. 1969.

AUERBACH-RUBIN, FRAN & OTTOLENGHI-NIGHTINGALE, ELENA: Effect of ethanol on the clearance of airborne pneumococci and the rate of pneumococcal transformations in the lung. *Infect. Immun.* 3:688–693, 1971.

AYERS, JOYCE; RUFF, CAROL F. & TEMPLER, DONALD I.: Alcoholism, cigarette smoking, coffee drinking and extraversion. *J. Stud. Alcohol* **37**: 983–985, 1976.

BANNER, ARTHUR S.: Pulmonary function in chronic alcoholism. *Am. Rev. Respir. Dis.* **108**:851–857, 1973.

BARRACLOUGH, B. M.: Poisoning cases: suicide or accident. *Br. J. Psychiatry* **124**:526–530, 1974.

BERFENSTAM, RAGNAR; LAGENBERG, DAGMAR & SMEDBY, BJÖRN: Victim characteristics in fatal home accidents. *Acta Socio-medica Scandinavica* **1**:145–164, 1969.

BESKOW, JAN: "Tveksamhet" – ett problem vid klassifikation av självmord. (Doubt – a problem when classifying suicide.) *Läkartidningen* **71**:2733–2734, 1974.

BINGHAM, J. R.: Precipitating factors in peptic ulcer. *Can. Med. Assoc. J.* **83**: 205–211, 1960.

BOLANDER, ANNE-MARIE: *Comparative study of mortality by cause in four Nordic countries, 1966–1968, with special reference to male excess mortality.* Statistiska Centralbyrån, SCB Statistical Reports Be 1971:9, Stockholm 1971.

BOWDEN, KEITH M. & MC CALLUM, NORMAN E. W.: Blood alcohol content: some aspects of its post-mortem uses. *Med. J. Aust.* **2**:36:78–81, 1949.

BRAYTON, ROBERT G.; STOKES, PETER E.; SCHWARTZ, MELVIN S. & LOURIA, DONALD B.: Effect of alcohol and various diseases on leukocyte mobilization, phagocytosis and intracellular bacterial killing. *N. Engl. J. Med.* **282**:123–128, 1970.

BRENNER, BERTHOLD: Alcoholism and fatal accidents. *Q. J. Stud. Alcohol* **28**:517–528, 1967.

BRUUN, KETTIL: *Alkoholi: käyttö, vaikutukset ja kontrolli* (Alcohol: use, effects and control). Tammi, Helsinki 1972.

BRUUN, KETTIL; EDWARDS, GRIFFITH; LUMIO, MARTTI; MÄKELÄ, KLAUS; PAN, LYNN; POPHAM, ROBERT E.; ROOM, ROBIN; SCHMIDT, WOLFGANG; SKOG, OLE-JØRGEN; SULKUNEN, PEKKA & ÖSTERBERG, ESA: *Alcohol control policies in public health perspective.* The Finnish Foundation for Alcohol Studies vol. 25, Forssa 1975.

BSCHOR, F.: Fettleber und Fettembolie. *Dtsch. Med. Wochenschr.* **88**:1112–1113, 1963.

BURCH, G. E.; HARB, J. M.; COLCOLOUGH, H. L. & TSUI, C. Y.: The effect of prolonged consumption of beer, wine and ethanol on the myocardium of the mouse. *Johns Hopkins Med. J.* **129**:130–148, 1971.

BURCH, GEORGE E. & GILES, THOMAS D.: Alcoholic cardiomyopathy. Pp. 435–460 in *The biology of alcoholism,* volume 3; *Clinical pathology,* eds. Benjamin Kissin & Henri Begleiter. Plenum press, New York 1974.

CHRISTOFFERSEN, PER & NIELSEN, KNUD: Histological changes in human liver biopsies from chronic alcoholics. *Acta Pathol. Microbiol. Scand.* (A) **80**:557–565, 1972.

COLLETT, JOHN: Nordisk alkoholstatistik 1971 (Nordic alcohol statistics 1971). *Alkoholfrågan* **66**:224–229, 1972.

CONWAY, NEVILLE: Haemodynamic effects of ethyl alcohol in patients with coronary heart disease. *Br. Heart J.* **30**:638–644, 1968.

COSTELLO, RAYMOND M. & SCHNEIDER, SANDRA LEE: Mortality in an alcoholic cohort. *Int. J. Addict.* **9**:355–363, 1974.

CRAVEY, ROBERT H. & JAIN, NARESH C.: Current status of blood alcohol methods. *Journal of chromatographic science* **12**:209–213, 1974.

DAVIS, GUSTAVE L.: Postmortem alcohol analyses of general aviation pilot fatalities. Armed forces institute of pathology 1962–67. *Aerospace Med.* **44**:80–83, 1973.

DAVIS, JOSEPH H.: Alcohol as a precursor to violent death. *J. Drug Issues* **5**:270–275, 1975.

DIDERICHSEN, AGNETE & SKYUM-NIELSEN, SVEND: *Om brug og misbrug af alkohol* (On the use and misuse of alcohol). Socialforskningsinstituttet, publikation 36, København 1969.

DIEM, K. & LENTNER, C. (eds.): *Scientific tables.* Seventh Edition. Ciba-Geigy limited, Basle 1973.

DUNDEE, JOHN W.; ISAAC, MARTIN; DAVIS, ELISABETH A. & SHERIDAN, BRIAN: Effects of rapid infusion of ethanol on some factors controlling blood sugar levels in man. *Q. J. Stud. Alcohol* **33**:722–733, 1972.

DURLACHER, STANLEY H.; MEIER, J. RALPH; FISHER, RUSSEL S. & LOVITT JR., WILLIAM W.: Sudden death due to pulmonary fat embolism in persons with alcoholic fatty liver. *Am. J. Pathol.* **30**:633–634, 1954.

EDGREN, CHRISTIAN & WIMAN, RONALD: *Suomalainen siirtolaistyövoima Ruotsissa vuonna 1972* (Finnish migrant labour force in Sweden in 1972). Elinkeinoelämän tutkimuslaitoksen julkaisuja C 3, Helsinki 1973. Moniste (Mimeographed).

EDMONDSON, HUGH A.; HALL, ERNEST M. & MYERS, RICHARD O.: Pathology of alcoholism. Pp. 233–290 in *Alcoholism,* ed. George N. Thompson. Charles C. Thomas, Springfield, Ill. 1956.

EMIRGIL, CEMIL; SOBOL, BRUCE J.; HEYMAN, BERNARD & SHIBUTANI, KINICHI: Pulmonary function in alcoholics. *Am. J. Med.* **57**:69–77, 1974.

ETTLINGER, RUTH W. & FLORDH, PER: Attempted suicide: experience of five hundred cases at a general hospital. *Acta Psychiatr. Scand.* Suppl. 103, 1955.

FALCONER, BERTIL & FALCONER, CHRIS: Postmortal blood alcohol in various parts of the vascular system. *Blutalkohol* **10**:328–335, 1973.

FATTEH, ABDULLAH & HAYES, BILL: Poisons that killed: an analysis of 300 cases. *N. C. Med. J.* **35**: 227–229, 1974.

FEINMAN, LAWRENCE & LIEBER, CHARLES S.: Liver disease in alcoholism. Pp. 303–338 in *The biology of alcoholism,* volume 3; *Clinical pathology,* eds. Benjamin Kissin & Henri Begleiter. Plenum press, New York 1974.

FISCHER, ERNST & WALLGREN HENRIK: Cerebral blood flow and cerebral alcohol uptake of anesthetized dogs. *Physiologist* **1**:27–28, 1957.

FORNEY, ROBERT B. & HARGER, R. N.: The alcohols. Pp. 210–231 in *Drill's pharmacology in medicine,* ed. J. R. DiPalma. McGraw-Hill, New York 1965.

FORNEY, ROBERT B. & HUGHES, FRANCIS W.: *Combined effects of alcohol and other drugs.* Charles C. Thomas, Springfield, Ill. 1968.

FORSANDER, O. & SUOMALAINEN, HEIKKI: Alcohol intake and erythrocyte aggregation. *Q. J. Stud. Alcohol* **16**:614–618, 1955.

FORSANDER, O.; VARTIA, K. O. & KRUSIUS, F.-E.: Experimentelle Studien über die biologische Wirkung von Alkohol. 1. Alkohol und Blutzucker. *Ann. Med. Exp. Biol. Fenn.* **36**:416–423, 1958.

FORSMAN, HEIKKI K.; GINMAN, LEIF & HIRVISALO, EVA L.: The blood ethanol level in patients taken into a psychiatric emergency ward. P. 34 in *Sixth Scandinavian meeting in Forensic Medicine.* Program and abstracts, June 16–18, Helsinki 1976.

FRANCISCO, J. T. & BALWIN, THOMAS EDWARD: Are post mortem alcohols valid? *Med. Times* **100**: 145–155, 1972.

FRENCH, SAMUEL W.: Acute and chronic toxicity of alcohol. Pp. 437–511 in *The biology of alcoholism,* volume 1; *Biochemistry,* eds. Benjamin Kissin & Henri Begleiter, Plenum press, New York 1971.

FREINKEL, NORBERT; ARKY, RONALD A.; SINGER, DAVID L.; COHEN, ALEX K.; BLEICHER, SHELDON J.; ANDERSON, JOHN B.; SILBERT, CYNTHIA K. & FOSTER, ANGELA E.: Alcohol hypoglycemia IV: current concepts of its pathogenesis. *Diabetes* **14**:350–361, 1965.

FREINKEL, NORBERT; SINGER, DAVID L.; ARKY, RONALD A.; BLEICHER, SHELDON J.; ANDERSON, JOHN B. & SILBERT, CYNTHIA K.: Alcohol hypoglycemia I: carbohydrate metabolism of patients with clinical alcohol hypoglycemia and the experimental reproduction of the syndrome with pure alcohol. *J. Clin. Invest.* **42**:1112–1133, 1963.

FRIBERG, LARS; CEDERLÖF, RUNE; LORICH, ULLA; LUNDMAN, TORBJÖRN;

& de FAIRE, ULF: Mortality in twins in relation to smoking habits and alcohol problems. *Arch. Environ. Health* 27:294–304, 1973.

FRIEDMAN, GARY D.; SIEGELAUB, A. B. & SELTZER, CARL C.: Cigarettes, alcohol, coffee and peptic ulcer. *N. Engl. Med.* **290**:469–473, 1974.

GIFFORD, HOUGHTON & TURKEL, HENRY W.: Diffusion of alcohol through stomach wall after death. *JAMA* **161**:866–868, 1956.

GOLDBERG, LEONARD.: *Quantitative studies on alcohol tolerance in man. The influence of ethyl alcohol on sensory, motor and psychological functions referred to blood alcohol in normal and habituated individuals.* Acta Physiol. Scand. **5**: Suppl. 16, 1943.

GORMSEN, HARALD: Retsmedicin (Forensic medicine). F.A.D.L.s Forlag, Århus 1973.

GOULD, LAWRENCE; REDDY, C. V. RAMANA; GOSWAMI, KUMAR; VENKATARAMAN, KALYANASUNDARAM & GOMPRECHT, ROBERT F.: Cardiac effects of two cocktails in normal man. *Chest* **63**:943–947, 1973.

GOULD, LAWRENCE; ZAHIR, MOHAMMAD; DE MARTINO, ANTHONY; GOMPRECHT, ROBERT F. & JAYNAL, FRANCIS: Hemodynamic effects of ethanol in patients with cardiac disease. *Q. J. Stud. Alcohol* 33:714–721, 1972.

GREEN, GARETH M. & KASS, EDWARD H.: Factors influencing the clearance of bacteria by the lung. *J. Clin. Invest.* **43**:769–776, 1964.

GÜRTLER, HANS & LUND, ALF: Sammenhæng mellem alkoholpåvirkethed og blodalkoholkoncentration hos trafikanter (Relationship between intoxication and blood alcohol concentration in subjects in traffic). *Ugeskr. Læger* **128**:1–15, 1966.

HABERMAN, PAUL W. & BADEN, MICHAEL M.: Alcoholism and violent death. *Q. J. Stud. Alcohol* 35:221–231, 1974.

HAGGARD, HOWARD W.; GREENBERG, LEON A. & RAKIETEN, NATHAN: Studies on the absorption, distribution and elimination of alcohol VI. *J. Pharmacol. Exp. Ther.* **69**:252–262, 1940.

HAMMOND, KEITH B.; RUMACK, BARRY H. & RODGERSON, DENIS O.: Blood ethanol – a report of unusually high levels in a living patient. *JAMA* 226:63–64, 1973.

HARENKO, AARNO: Alkohol och suicidförsök genom förgiftning i Helsingfors åren 1962–64. (Alcohol and attempted suicide by poisoning in Helsinki in 1962–64). *Sosiaalilääketieteellinen aikakauslehti* 6:27–31, 1968.

HIMWICH, HAROLD E.: The physiology of alcohol. *JAMA* **163**: 545–549, 1957.

HOGNESTAD, JENS & TEISBERG, PER: Heart pathology in chronic alcoholism. *Acta Pathol. Microbiol. Scand.* (A) **81**:315–322, 1973.

HOLLANDER, M. & WOLFE, D. A.: *Nonparametric statistical methods.* Wiley J. & Sons, New York 1973.

HOWARD, JOHN M. & EHRLICH, EDWARD W.: A clinical study of alcoholic pancreatitis. *Surg. Gynecol. Obstet.* 113:167–173, 1961.

HOVE, HARALD: Reddede selvmordspatienters skæbne (The fate of saved suicidal patients). *Ugeskr. Læger* 155:645–646, 1953.

HUBER, OSWALD: Über die Diffusion des Äthylalkohols in menschlichen Leichen. *Dtsch. Z. Ges. Gerichtl. Med.* 37:128–135, 1943.

HUHTALA, A.: Kuolemaan johtaneista etyyli- ja metyylialkoholimyrkytyksistä Suomessa vuosina 1936–49 (Fatal ethyl- and methyl alcohol poisonings in Finland in the years 1936–49.). *Alkoholiliikkeen aikakauskirja* 3:53–62, 1951 (osa I) & 3:109–115, 1951 (osa II).

HUSS, M.: *Alcoholismus chronicus eller chronisk alkoholsjukdom* (Alcoholismus chronicus or chronic alcoholic disease). Joh. Beckman, Stockholm 1849.

HÄLLÉN, J. & KROOK, H.: Follow-up studies on an unselected ten-year material of 360 patients with liver cirrhosis in one community. *Acta Med. Scand.* 173:479–493, 1963.

HÄRTEL, GOTTFRIED; LOUHIJA, ANTTI; KONTTINEN, AARNE & WESTLING, ACHILLES: Alkoholistien kliiniset sydän- ja laboratoriolöydökset (Cardiovascular and laboratory findings in chronic alcoholics). *Duodecim* 85: 740–745, 1969.

HÄUSSLER, MICHAEL & MALLACH, HANS JOACHIM: Weitere Betrachtungen über Blutalkoholwerte über 3 Promille. *Blutalkohol* 10: 159–165, 1973.

IRGENS-JENSEN, OLAV: *Alkoholvaner i en utkantkommune* (Alcohol habits in a remote community). Universitetsforlaget, Oslo 1965.

ISOTALO, ANTTI: Lääkärin tehtävät kuolemantapauksessa (The physician's duties in connection with deaths). Pp. 131–134 in *Oikeuslääketiede* (Forensic medicine), ed. Unto Uotila. WSOY, Porvoo 1970.

IVY, A. C. & GIBBS, E. G.: Pancreatitis: a review. *Surgery* 31:614–642, 1952.

JACOBSON, NILS-OLOF & ERIKSSON, JOHN-OLOF: T-spritmissbruket – ett tilltagande problem (Misuse of T-spirits – a growing problem). *Socialmedicinsk tidskrift* 3:201–205, 1972.

JAKOBSSON, STEN V.: *Forensic medicine in Sweden 1973*. Paper presented at the Annual Meeting of Forensic Sciences in New York, April 1973.

JAROSCH, K.: Interpretation höherer Blutalkoholwerte. *Blutalkohol* 12:192–203, 1975.

JELLINEK, E. M.: *The disease concept of alcoholism.* Hillhouse press, New Haven 1960.

JOKIPII, S. G.: *Experimental studies on blood alcohol in healthy subjects and in some diseases.* Ann. Med. Exp. Biol. Fenn. 29: Suppl. 2, Helsinki 1951.

KAGER, LARS; LINDBERG, STAFFAN & ÅGREN, GUNNAR: Alcohol consumption and acute pancreatitis in men. *Scand. J. Gastroenterol.* 7: Suppl. 15, 1972.

KALANT, H.: Interpretation of post-mortem ethanol concentrations. *Aerospace Med.* 39:633–637, 1968.

KALANT, H.: Pharmacological and behavioral variables in the development of alcohol tolerance. Pp. 44–55 in *Pharmacology and the future of man.* Proc. 5th Int. Congr. Pharmacology, San Francisco 1972, vol. 1. Karger, Basel 1973.

KARU, ELMAR: Bemerkungen zur Einleitung der Blutalkoholkurve. *Blutalkohol* 12:307–315, 1975.

KASTENGREN, CLAES: Förgiftningar med dödlig utgång i Malmö (Fatal poisonings in Malmö). *Läkartidningen* **71**:1742–1744, 1974.

KATER, RODERICK M. H.; CARULLI, NICOLA & IBER, FRANK L.: Differences in the rate of ethanol metabolism in recently drinking alcoholic and nondrinking subjects. *Am. J. Clin. Nutr.* 22:1608–1617, 1969.

KAYE, SIDNEY & HAAG, HARVEY B.: Terminal blood alcohol concentrations in ninety-four fatal cases of acute alcoholism. *JAMA* **165**:451–452, 1957.

KEROSUO, MARTTI: Alkoholismin levinneisyys Suomessa (Prevalence of alcoholism in Finland). *Alkoholipolitiikka* 35:78–85, 1970.

KLEPSER, R. G. & NUNGESTER, W. J.: The effect of alcohol upon the chemotactic response of leucocytes. *J. Infect. Dis.* **65**:196–199, 1939.

KLINGMAN, GERDA I. & HAAG, HARVEY B.: Studies on severe alcohol intoxication in dogs. *Q. J. Stud. Alcohol* **19**:203–225, 1958.

Korvikealkoholitoimikunnan osamietintö (Partial report of the committee on substitute alcohols). Kom.miet. 1973:53, Helsinki 1973.

KOPPANYI, T.; CANARY, J. J. & MAENGWYN-DAVIES, G. D.: Problems in acute alcohol poisoning. *Q. J. Stud. Alcohol* **22**: Suppl. 1:24–36, 1961.

KOSSMAN, KARL THEODOR: Das Vorkommen von Blutalkoholkonzentrationen über 3 Promille bei Verkehrsstraftätern. *Blutalkohol* **9**:486–488, 1972.

KRAMER, KARL; KULLER, LEWIS & FISHER, RUSSEL: The increasing mortality attributed to cirrhosis and fatty liver in Baltimore (1957–1966). *Ann. Intern. Med.* **69**:273–282, 1968.

KULLER, LEWIS; LILIENFELD, ABRAHAM & FISHER, RUSSEL: Sudden and unexpected deaths in young adults. *JAMA* **198**:248–252, 1966.

KYÖSOLA, KIMMO & FOCK, GUSTAF: Pankreatiitti (Pancreatitis). *Duodecim* **89**:905–913, 1973.

LAURENZI, GUSTAVE A. & GUARNERI, JOSEPH J.: A study of the mechanisms of pulmonary resistance to infection: the relationship of bacterial clearance to ciliary and alveolar macrophage function. *Am. Rev. Respir. Dis.* **93**: Suppl.: 134–141, 1966.

LAW, DENNIS K.; DUDRICK, STANLEY J. & ABDOU, NABIH I.: Immunocompetence of patients with protein-calorie malnutrition. The effects of nutritional repletion. *Ann. Intern. Med.* **79**:545–550, 1973.

LELBACH, WERNER K.: Organic pathology related to volume and pattern of alcohol use. Pp. 93–198 in *Research advances in alcohol and drug problems,* volume 1, eds. Robert J. Gibbins, Yedy Israel, Harold Kalant, Robert E. Popham, Wolfgang Schmidt & Reginald G. Smart. John Wiley & Sons, New York 1974.

LEVY, LEONARD J.; DUGA, JUDITH; GIRGIS, MEDHAT & GORDON, EDWIN E.: Ketoacidosis associated with alcoholism in nondiabetic subjects. *Ann. Intern. Med.* **78**:213–219, 1973.

LIEBER, C. S.; SPRITZ, N. & DE CARLI, L. M.: Accumulation of triglycerides in heart and kidney after alcohol ingestion (abstract). *J. Clin. Invest.* **45**: 1041, 1966.

LIEBER, CHARLES S.: Alcohol and the liver: transition from metabolic adaptation to tissue injury and cirrhosis. Pp. 171–188 in *Alcoholic liver pathology,* eds. J. M. Khanna, Y. Israel & H. Kalant. Alcoholism and Drug Addiction Research Foundation of Ontario, Toronto 1975.

LINCK, KONRAD: Alter, letale Dosis und Blutalkoholbefunde bei der tödlichen Aethylalkoholvergiftung. *Med. Klin.* **18**:570–572, 1950.

LINCK, KONRAD: Blut-, Urin- und Liquoralkoholkurve des Menschen bei akuter Alkoholvergiftung und der Zeitpunkt des Todeseintritts. *Z. Gerichl. Med.* **39**:514–528, 1948/49.

LINCK, KONRAD: Zum Problem der akuten tödlichen Alkoholvergiftung. *Fortschr. Med.* **71**:183–184, 1953.

LINDFORS, KAJ -OLOF: Finnish immigrants in psychiatric care in Sweden. *Acta Psychiatr. Scand.,* **53**: Suppl. 265:29, 1976.

LIU, YONG K.: Leukopenia in alcoholics. *Am. J. Med.* **54**:605–610, 1973.

LOOMIS, TED A.: The effect of alcohol on myocardial and respiratory function. *Q. J. Stud. Alcohol* **13**:561–570, 1952.

LORBER, STANLEY H.; DINOSO, VICENTE P. & CHEY, WILLIAM Y.: Diseases of the gastrointestinal tract. Pp. 339–357 in *The biology of alcoholism,* volume 3; *Clinical pathology,* eds. Benjamin Kissin & Henri Begleiter. Plenum press, New York 1974.

LOUHIJA, ANTTI: Alkoholin kardiovaskulaariset vaikutukset (Cardiovascular effects of alcohol). *Duodecim* **88**:292–299, 1972.

LOURIA, DONALD B.: Susceptibility to infection during experimental alcohol intoxication. *Trans. Assoc. Am. Physicians* **76**:102–112, 1963.

LUNDEVALL, JON: *Rettsmedisin* (Forensic medicine). Universitetsforlaget, Oslo 1973.

LUNDH, G.: Pankreatit – nya synpunkter på etiologi, diagnostik och behandling (Pancreatitis – new aspects of etiology, diagnostics and treatment). *Nord. Med.* **84**:1353–1359, 1970.

LYNCH, MATTHEW J. G.; RAPHAEL, STANLEY & DIXON, THOMAS P.: Fat embolism in chronic alcoholism. *Arch. Pathol.* **67**:68–80, 1959.

LÖNNQVIST, JOUKO: *Suicide in Helsinki. An epidemiological and social-psychiatric study of suicides in Helsinki in 1960–61 and 1970–71.* Monographs of Psychiatria Fennica No. 8, Helsinki 1977.

MC BAY, ARTHUR J. & HUDSON, PAGE: Drug deaths in North Carolina: a brief survey of deaths attributed to drugs in North Carolina 1973. *N. C. Med. J.* **35**:542–544, 1974.

MADISON, LEONARD L.: Ethanol-induced hypoglycemia. Pp. 85–107 in *Advances in metabolic disorders,* volume 3, eds. R. Levine & R. Lufts. Academic Press, London 1968.

MADISON, LEONARD L.; LOCHNER, AMANDA & WULFF, JOHAN: Ethanol induced hypoglycemia. *Diabetes* **16**:252–258, 1967.

MAJCHROWICZ, EDWARD & MENDELSON, JACK H.: Blood methanol concentrations during experimentally induced ethanol intoxication in alcoholics. *J. Pharmacol. Exp. Ther.* **179**:293–300, 1971.

MALEZKY, BARRY M. & KLOTTER, JAMES: Smoking and alcoholism. *Am. J. Psychiatry* **131**:445–447, 1974.

MARCINKOWSKI, TADEUSZ & PRYZYBYLSKI, ZYGMUNT: Evaluation of the cause of death in cases of acute alcohol poisoning. *Forensic Sci.* **4**:233–238, 1974.

MELLANBY, E.: Alcohol: its absorption into and disappearance from the blood under different conditions. Medical Research Committee, Special Report Series No. 31, His Majesty's Stationary Office, London 1919. Quoted in Wallgren, Henrik & Barry, Herbert, III: *Actions of alcohol,* volume I, p. 95. Elsevier Publishing Company, Amsterdam 1970.

MENDELSON, JACK H. & LA DOU, JOSEPH: Experimentally induced chronic intoxication and withdrawal in alcoholics. Part 2. Psychophysiological findings. *Q. J. Stud. Alcohol,* suppl. 2:14–39, 1964.

MEZEY, ESTEBAN: Blood alcohol. *JAMA* **227**:441, 1974.

MEZEY, ESTEBAN & TOBON, FABIO: Rates of ethanol clearance and activities of the ethanol-oxidizing enzymes in chronic alcoholic patients. *Gastroenterology* **61**:707–715, 1971.

MOSKOW, HERBERT A.; PENNINGTON, RAYMOND C. & KNISELY, MELVIN H.: Alcohol, sludge and hypoxic areas of nervous system, liver and heart. *Microvasc. Res.* **1**:174–185, 1968.

MURTO, LASSE: *Asunnottomien alkoholistien yhteiskuntaan paluun vaikeudet* (Problems connected with return to society among alcoholics with no fixed abode). Tampereen yliopiston sosiaalipolitiikan laitoksen tutkimuksia 27, Tampere 1972. Moniste (Mimeographed).

MYRHED, MÅRTEN: *Alcohol consumption in relation to factors associated with ischemic heart disease.* Acta Med. Scand. Suppl. 567, 1974.

MÖSSLACHER, H.: Die Alkoholkardiomyopathie. *Wien. Klin. Wochenschr.* **10**: Suppl. 1:3–22, 1973.

Nordic Council: *Yearbook of Nordic statistics 1971.* (10th edition), Stockholm 1972.

NUNGESTER, W. J. & KLEPSER, R. G.: A possible mechanism of lowered resistance to pneumonia. *J. Infect. Dis.* 63:94–102, 1938.

Oikeuslääketieteellisten ruumiinavausten järjestelyä selvittävän toimikunnan mietintö (Report of the committee on the organization of medicolegal autopsies). Kom. miet. 1971: B 49, Helsinki 1971.

O'TOOLE, WILLIAM F.; SAXENA, HARI M. K.; GOLDEN, ABNER & RITTS, ROY E.: Studies of postmortem microbiology using sterile autopsy technique. *Arch. Pathol.* 80:540–547, 1965.

PACHINGER, OTHAR M.; TILLMANNS, HARALD; MAO, JAMES C.; FAUVEL, JEAN-MARIE & BING, RICHARD J.: The effects of prolonged administration of ethanol on cardiac metabolism and performance in the dog. *J. Clin. Invest.* 52:2690–2696, 1973.

PAFFENBARGER, RALPH S. JR.; WING, ALVIN L. & HYDE, ROBERT T.: Chronic disease in former college students XIII. Early precursors of peptic ulcer. *Am. J. Epidemiol.* 100:307–315, 1974.

PALMER, EDDY: Gastritis: a re-evaluation. *Medicine* 33:199–290, 1954.

PAWAN, G. L. S.: Metabolism of alcohol (ethanol) in man. *Proc. Nutr. Soc.* 31:83–89, 1972.

PENNINGTON, RAYMOND C. & KNISELY, MELVIN H.: Experiments aimed at separating the mechanical circulatory effects of ethanol from specific chemical effects. *Ann. N. Y. Acad. Sci.* 215:356–365, 1973.

PENTTILÄ, A.; TENHU, M. & KATAJA, M.: Das Vorkommen von hohem Blutalkoholgehalt (über 3 o/oo) bei im Strassenverkehr angetroffenen Personen. *Blutalkohol* 9:45–52, 1972.

PLUECKHAHN, V. D. & BALLARD, B.: Diffusion of stomach alcohol and heart blood alcohol concentration at autopsy. *J. Forensic Sci.* 12:463–470, 1967.

PLUECKHAHN, VERNON D.: The evaluation of autopsy blood alcohol levels. *Med. Sci. Law* 8:168–176, 1968.

PLUECKHAHN, VERNON D.: The significance of blood alcohol levels at autopsy. *Med. J. Aust.* 2:54:118–124, 1967.

POIKOLAINEN, K.; KIVIRANTA, P. & SUOMINEN, J.: Alcoholism and work-disability pensions in Finland. Pp. 291–297 in *Psychiatria Fennica 1973.* The Psychiatric Clinic of the Helsinki University Central Hospital, Helsinki 1973.

POLACZEK-KORNECKI, T.; ZELAZNY, T.; WALCZAK, Z.; DENDURA, S. & SZPAK, E.: Experimentelle Untersuchungen über den Todesmechanismus bei akuter Alkoholvergiftung. Die Rolle der Ateminsuffizienz. *Anaesthesist* 21:266–270, 1971.

PROKOP, O.: *Forensische Medizin.* VEB Verlag Volk und Gesundheit. Berlin 1966.

PUFFER, R. R. & GRIFFITH, G. W.: *Patterns of urban mortality*. Pan American Health Organization, Scientific publication No. 151, Washington D. C. 1967.

PÖYSÄ, TOIVO & MÄKELÄ, KLAUS: Korvikealkoholin juopottelukäyttö ennen ja jälkeen lainuudistuksen (The use of substitute alcohol as an intoxicant before and after the revision of law). *Alkoholipolitiikka* 6:3–7, 1970.

RANKIN, J. G.; HALE, G. S.; WILKINSON, P.; O'DAY, D. M.; SANTAMARIA, J. N. & BABARCZY, G.: Relationship between smoking and pulmonary disease in alcoholism. *Med. J. Aust.* 1:56:730–733, 1969.

REGAN, TIMOTHY J.; KHAN, MOHAMMAD I.; ETTINGER, PHILIP O.; HAIDER, BUNYAD; LYONS, MICHAEL M. & OLDEWURTEL, HENRY A.: Myocardial function and lipid metabolism in the chronic alcoholic animal. *J. Clin. Invest.* **54**:740–752, 1974.

REGAN, TIMOTHY J.; KOROXENIDIS, GABRIEL; MOSCHOS, CHRISTOS B.; OLDEWURTEL, HENRY A.; LEHAN, PATRICK H. & HELLEMS, HARPER K.: The acute metabolic and hemodynamic responses of the left ventricle to ethanol. *J. Clin. Invest.* **45**:270–280, 1966.

REGAN, TIMOTHY J.; LEVINSON, GILBERT E.; OLDEWURTEL, HENRY A.; FRANK, MARTIN J.; WEISSE, ALLEN B. & MOSCHOS, CHRISTOS B.: Ventricular function in noncardiacs with alcoholic fatty liver: role of ethanol in the production of cardiomyopathy. *J. Clin. Invest.* **48**:397–407, 1969.

REGUS, FRITZ: Akute Alkoholvergiftung mit Todesfolge. *Sammlung von Vergiftungsfällen* **8**:119–130 (A 688), 1937.

REISBY, NILS: Den inter- og intraindividuelle variation af blodalkoholkoncentrationen hos normale forsøgspersoner (The inter- and intraindividual variation of blood alcohol concentrations in normal test subjects. *Ugeskr. Læger* **133**:139–143, 1971.

REMINGTON, RICHARD & SCHORK, M. ANTHONY: *Statistics with applications to the biological and health sciences*. Prentice-Hall Inc., Englewood Cliffs, New Jersey 1970.

RODIER, J. & GENTILE, F.: Intoxication alcoolique aiguë. *Maroc. Med.* **31**: 806–807, 1952.

ROSENSTEIN, R.; MC CARTHY, L. & BORISON, H. L.: Respiratory effects of ethanol and procaine injected into the cerebrospinal fluid of the brainstem in cats. *J. Pharmacol. Exp. Ther.* **162**:174–181, 1968.

SALDEEN, T.: *Kursen i rättsmedicin* (The curriculum in forensic medicine). Uppsala sine data. Stencil (Mimeographed).

SALDEEN, TOM & JOHANSSON, ÖRIAN: The significance of chronic heart disease, fatty liver and consumption of barbiturate and librium on the tolerance to ethyl alcohol, as judged in a postmortem series. *J. Forensic Sci.* 12:273–294, 1967.

SALUM, INNA (ed.): *Delirium tremens and certain other acute sequels of alcohol abuse.* Acta Psychiatr. Scand., Suppl. 235, Stockholm 1972.

SARIOLA, SAKARI: *Drinking patterns in Finnish Lapland.* The Finnish Foundation of Alcohol Studies, Helsinki 1956.

SARLES, H. & TISCORNIA, O.: Ethanol and chronic calcifying pancreatitis. *Med. Clin. North Am.* 58:1333–1346, 1974.

SCHERRER-ETIENNE, M. & POSTERNAK, J. M.: Pénétration et répartition de l'éthanol et du pentobarbital dans le cerveau du chat. *Schweiz. Med. Wochenschr.* 93:1016–1020, 1963.

SCHMIDT, WOLFGANG & DE LINT, JAN: Causes of death of alcoholics. *Q. J. Stud. Alcohol* 33:171–185, 1972.

SEVITT, SIMON: The significance and classification of fat-embolism. *Lancet* 2: 825–828, 1960.

SHAH, MADHUKAR N.; CLANCY, BARBARA A. & IBER, FRANK, L.: Comparison of blood clearance of ethanol and tolbutamide and the activity of hepatic ethanol-oxidizing and drug-metabolizing enzymes in chronic alcoholic subjects. *Am. J. Clin. Nutr.* 25:135–139, 1972.

SJÖBERG, LARS: Beräkningssätt i fråga om alkoholhalt och förbränning (Calculation methods for alcohol concentration and oxidation). *Alkoholfrågan* 58:317–327, 1964.

Socialstyrelsen: Socialstyrelsens circulär med råd och anvisningar angående dödsbevis; den 14 maj 1971 (Circular letter by the National Board of Social Affairs on the issuing of death certificates; the 14th of May 1971). Nr 24, Stockholm 1971.

SPIEGEL, MURRAY R.: *Statistics.* Schaum's outline series. Mc-Graw-Hill, United States 1961.

SPRADLEY, JAMES P.: *You owe yourself a drunk.* Little, Brown and Company, Boston 1970.

STILLMAN, ERNEST G.: Persistence of inspired bacteria in the lungs of alcoholized mice. *J. Exp. Med.* 40:353–361, 1924.

SUNDBY, PER: *Alcoholism and mortality.* Universitetsforlaget, Oslo 1967.

SUNSHINE, IRVING & HODNETT, NICHOLAS: Methods for the determination of ethanol and acetaldehyde. Pp. 545–573 in *The biology of alcoholism,* volume 1; *Biochemistry,* eds. Benjamin Kissin & Henri Begleiter. Plenum Press, New York 1971.

SVENDSEN, HANS OLE: Mortaliteten af levercirrose og forbruget af alkohol i nordiske lande 1961–1972 (The mortality from cirrhosis of the liver and alcohol consumption in the Scandinavian countries in 1961–1972). *Ugeskr. Læger* 138:1901–1905, 1976.

THALER, H.: Schlusswort. *Dtsch. Med. Wochenschr.* 88:1113, 1963.

TISMAN, GLENN & HERBERT, VICTOR: In vitro myelosuppression and immunosuppression by ethanol. *J. Clin. Invest.* 52:1410–1414, 1973.

UGARTE, GUILLERMO; PEREDA, TAMARA; PINO, MARIA EUGENIA & ITURRIAGA, HERNÁN: Influence of alcohol intake, length of abstinence and meprobamate on the rate of ethanol metabolism in man. *Q. J. Stud. Alcohol* 33:698–705, 1972.

WADMAN, BENGT; SPENCER, EDWIN & WERNER, IVAR: Liver cirrhosis in three Scandinavian communities: an attempt at a critical evaluation of available epidemiologic data. *Acta Med. Scand.* **189**:221–230, 1971.

WALLGREN, HENRIK & BARRY, HERBERT, III: *Actions of alcohol,* I–II. Elsevier Publishing Company, Amsterdam 1970.

WEILER, G. & REH, H.: Der Beweiswert gaschromatographischer Blutalkoholbestimmungen bei Leichenfäulnis. *Blutalkohol* 11:402–408, 1974.

WEINER, H. A. & TENNANT, ROBERT: A statistical study of acute hemorrhagic pancreatitis (hemorrhagic necrosis of pancreas). *Am. J. Med. Sci.* **196**:167–176, 1938.

WIDMARK, E. M. P.: *Die teoretischen Grundlagen und die praktische Verwendbarkeit der gerichtlich-medizinischen Alkoholbestimmung.* Urban & Schwartzenberg, Berlin 1932.

WIDMARK, ERIK M. P.: Die Maximalgrenzen der Alkoholkonsumption. *Biochem. Z.* 259:285–293, 1933.

WOLTHERS, HENNING: *Undersøgelser over postmortel alkoholdannelse* (Studies on postmortal alcohol formation). Christtreus bogtrykkeri. København 1958.

World Health Organization: *Manual of the international statistical classification of diseases, injuries, and causes of death* (The Seventh Revision), Vol. 1. Geneva 1957.

World Health Organization: *Manual of the international statistical classification of diseases, injuries, and causes of death* (The Eighth Revision), vol. 1. Geneva 1967.

ZINK, PETER & REINHARDT, GÜNTER: Zur Dauer der Resorptionphase. *Blutalkohol* 12:100–107, 1975.

SOURCES OF STATISTICAL DATA

Hagskýrslur Íslands II, 61. Mannfjöldaskýrslur árin 1961–1970. Hagstofu Íslands, Reykjavik, Ísland (Statistics of Iceland. Population and vital statistics 1961–1970. Statistical Bureau of Iceland, Reykjavik, Iceland).

Norges offisielle statistikk. Dødsårsaker 1961–1973. Statistisk sentralbyrå, Oslo, Norge (Official Statistics of Norway. Causes of Death 1961–1973. Central Bureau of Statistics of Norway, Oslo, Norway).

Sundhedsstyrelsen. Dødsårsagerne i Danmark 1961–1973. København, Danmark (National Health Service of Denmark. Causes of Death in the Kingdom of Denmark. Copenhagen, Denmark).

Suomen virallinen tilasto, sarja VI B. Kuolemansyyt 1961–1973, Tilastokeskus, Helsinki, Suomi – Finlands officiella statistik, serie VI B. Dödsorsaker 1961–1973, Helsingfors, Finland (Official Statistics of Finland, series VI B. Causes of Death in Finland 1961–1973. Central Statistical Office of Finland, Helsinki, Finland).

Sveriges officiella statistik. Dödsorsaker 1971–1973. Statistiska centralbyrån, Stockholm, Sverige (Official Statistics of Sweden. Causes of Death 1961–1973. National Central Bureau of Statistics, Stockholm, Sweden).

SOURCES OF STATISTICAL DATA

[illegible]